THE
knife's
edge

THE
knife's edge

The Heart and Mind of a Cardiac Surgeon

PROFESSOR
STEPHEN WESTABY

Certain details, including names, places and dates,
have been changed to protect privacy.

Mudlark
An imprint of HarperCollins*Publishers*
1 London Bridge Street
London SE1 9GF

www.harpercollins.co.uk

First published by Mudlark 2019

1 3 5 7 9 10 8 6 4 2

A catalogue record of this book is
available from the British Library

HB ISBN 978-0-00-828577-7
PB ISBN 978-0-00-828581-4

Printed and bound in Great Britain by
CPI (UK) Ltd, Croydon

MIX
Paper from
responsible sources
FSC™ C007454

For Sarah, who saved me from myself, together with Gemma and Mark, then Alice and Chloe, the children and grandchildren who give me so much pleasure.

contents

preface

EVERY SINGLE HEART OPERATION risks a life. This tension between kill or cure is unique to my specialty, with no professional equivalent, and few people can live with it on a daily basis. During my formative years, to operate within the heart was seen as the last surgical frontier. Direct vision repair was considered as difficult as landing on the moon or splitting the atom. Then the heart–lung machine and the swinging sixties changed everything. Heart transplants and artificial hearts both emerged during my impressionable medical school years. When I embarked on training in the 1970s, heart surgery remained an exclusive and remote club that was exceptionally difficult to join. Yet I was eventually granted the profound privilege of being able to improve thousands of lives.

Each heart is unique in its own way. Although most operations prove straightforward and uneventful, some evolve into an extraordinary battle for survival and a few are quite literally a bloody disaster. As my experience and knowledge increased, I became a last port of call for the cardiologically destitute, a depository for cases that no one else wanted, at home and abroad. Ultimately I lost patients whom I knew could be saved with equipment we were denied in the NHS. The recriminations that accompany death soon followed. An agonising interview with the bereaved, dismal discussions at the 'Morbidity and Mortality Meeting,' then a joyless visit to the coroner's court. I was vehemently outspoken about the system's deficiencies, and suffered as a result. The NHS doesn't care for those who do not conform.

In this book I have set out to describe how it felt to be a heart surgeon as the specialty emerged and what it is like in the current hostile environment. I have depicted the physical and the psychological endeavour, the emotional highs and lows, the triumphs and the disappointments, and how being a surgeon affected me and my loved ones. When I was a young man, as we shall see, a peculiar quirk of fate helped me by dispelling my inhibitions and rendering me immune to fear. It's not something I would freely recommend and it was a curious launchpad for a career at the sharp end, one that enabled me to embrace challenges that others would wish to avoid.

For someone who is not a professional writer, it takes an inordinate amount of time and effort to write a book for public consumption. You will undoubtedly conclude that I was more the surgeon than the literary genius, yet to my delight my first book, *Fragile Lives*, became an award-winning bestseller. As the title suggests, the book largely focused on remarkable cases. *The Knife's Edge* is darker. It describes my humble beginnings, my struggle to succeed, and my priceless relationships with some of the pioneers and great leaders of the specialty. Because of the huge risks involved and the pile of bodies that ensued, the pioneers all manifested a particular personality type – bold, determined, often flamboyant, with resilience and immunity to grief. Sadly, so taxing is the lifestyle that by the end of my career few UK graduates were prepared to make it their calling and career. The 'end of an era', or the 'end of the beginning' as some would put it.

The whole riveting story of modern heart surgery evolved during my lifetime, and I was proud to be part of it.

introduction

JUST WEEKS AFTER MY SURGICAL CAREER came to an end I was invited to present the prizes at a local school speech day. The headmistress urged me to treat the teenagers as adults, and suggested that I convey to them what personal qualities I possessed that enabled me to become a cardiac surgeon. By this stage I had a stock response: 'To study medicine,' I said to the assembled schoolchildren, 'demands an unstinting work ethic and great determination. Then it requires more than a modicum of manual dexterity, together with supreme confidence to train as a surgeon. To aspire to become a heart surgeon and risk a patient's life every time you operate is a step beyond. For that you need the courage to fail.'

This last phrase wasn't original – it was regularly used to describe the heart surgery pioneers in the era when more patients died than survived – but the kids didn't know that. I decided to omit the claim that gender, social class, colour and creed played no part, because I really didn't believe it myself. Nor did I regard myself as possessing all the qualities I talked about. I was more of an artist. My fingertips and brain were connected.

After rewarding the school swats, I started nonchalantly answering questions about my achievements in Oxford. With considerable insight, one biology boffin asked how it's possible to operate inside an organ that pumps five litres of blood every minute and whether the brain dies if the heart stops. Another wanted to know how to get to the heart when it's surrounded by ribs, breast-bone and spine. Then the art teacher asked what causes blue babies, as if someone paints them blue.

Coming to the end of the session, a bespectacled little girl with pigtails raised her hand. Standing up like a poppy in a cornfield, she boomed out, 'Sir, how many of your patients died?'

So loud was her earnest approach that there was no way I could pretend not to hear. One set of parents tried to disappear under the floorboards while the flustered headmistress began explaining that it was time for the honoured guest to now leave. But I couldn't ignore this inquisitive individual in front of her friends. I considered the question for a moment, then had to confess: 'I really don't know the answer to that. More than most soldiers but fewer than a bomber pilot, I guess.' At least fewer than *Enola Gay* over Hiroshima, I thought to myself cynically.

Quick as a flash, Miss Curiosity probed again. 'Can you remember them all? Did they make you sad?'

Another brief moment of deliberation. Could I admit to a hall full of parents, teachers and schoolchildren that

I had no idea exactly how many patients I had dispatched, let alone recall their names. I could only muster one response: 'Yes, every death upset me.' I waited to be struck down with a thunderbolt but mercifully that was the end of our brief dialogue.

It was only after I stopped being an inadvertent serial killer that I began to remember patients as people, rather than simply recalling mortality statistics and the many times I went along to autopsies or coroner's courts. And there were deaths that haunted me, not least the young people who succumbed needlessly to heart failure. Those who were not accepted for transplantation but who could have been saved with the new circulatory support devices that our NHS declined to pay for.

In the 1970s one in five of my boss's cases at the Brompton Hospital died after surgery. As a cocky trainee I would greet each patient, record their medical history, then listen to their fears and expectations about the upcoming operation. Most were severely symptomatic, having waited months to come to the famous hospital in London. It didn't take long for me to predict the ones who wouldn't make it, usually the ones with rheumatic valve disease who arrived in a wheelchair and could barely speak on account of their breathlessness. Breathlessness is uniquely terrifying, likened by the patient to drowning or suffocation. They didn't die because of poor needlework. They simply couldn't tolerate their time on the heart–lung machine or the poor protection afforded to heart muscle during surgery in those days. We all knew that the slower the surgeon, the more likely the patient was to die. We would take bets on it. 'If X does the valve replacement he stands a chance. But he's buggered with Y.'

That was the way it used to be in the NHS. Treatment was free, so the punters didn't question what was on offer. Life or death followed from the toss of the dice. But the finality of death was still devastating. The consultants would shield themselves from all the misery by dispatching us juniors to talk with the family.

I seldom had to speak. The bereaved relatives would recognise the slow walk with dropped shoulders and head down as I approached. They could read my unequivocal 'bad news' expression. After the reflex indrawing of breath came shock, my words 'Sorry' and 'Didn't make it' triggering emotional disintegration. The sudden relief of suspense and the subsequent crushing grief were often followed by dignified resignation, but sometimes by abject denial or frank meltdown. I've had hysterical demands for me to return to theatre and resurrect the corpse, to resume cardiac massage or put the body back on the bypass machine. It was particularly heart-breaking for the parents of young children, little ones who had just developed their own innocent personality. As I saw it, newborn babies just screamed and pooed, but toddlers were well on their way to becoming people. They walked in holding Mummy's hand and clutching their teddy bears, which all too often were carried off with them to the mortuary fridge. Yet the minute I turned and walked away from these families, my sorrow was filed in the out tray. Eventually, when I started to lose my own patients, I became well used to it.

Only once did it strike me that I had murdered some-one, and the grim circumstances came as a shocking and bloody reminder that I was not invincible. It was a third-time operation on the mitral valve of a middle-aged patient who had a huge heart on the chest X-ray and excessively high pressures in the right ventricle situated directly below the breast-bone. I always took precautions when reopening the chest after previous surgery, and had started to request a CT scan to determine the gap between bone and heart. This led to me being admonished for adding to the costs of my many reoperations – only committees were allowed to sanction additional expense. The gentleman's anxious partner accompanied him to the anaesthetic room and I urged her not to worry. I told her I was very experienced and would take good care of him.

'That's why we came to you,' she replied, her voice quivering with apprehension. She kissed his forehead and slipped out.

I drew the knife along the old scar and used the electro-cautery to singe the outer table of the sternum. The wire cutter snipped the steel wires from the second operation, which I then tore out with heavy grasping forceps. It was just like pulling teeth – should they break, it makes life difficult. The oscillating saw screeched against them as if screaming, 'I'm not designed to cut steel.' Then came the tricky bit, which involved edging my way through the full thickness of bone with a powerful saw designed not to lacerate the soft tissues beneath. I had safely reopened the sternum for hundreds of reoperations, but this time there was a great 'whoosh'. Dark blue blood hosed out through the slit in the bone, poured down my gown, splashed onto my clogs and streamed across the floor.

I let out a chain of expletives. While I pressed hard over the incision to slow the bleeding, I instructed my jelly-legged assistant to cannulate the blood vessels in the groin so we could get onto the bypass machine. As the anaesthetist frantically squeezed in bags of donor blood through the drips in the neck, it all went dreadfully wrong. The cannula dissected the layers of the main leg artery so we couldn't establish any flow. With continued profuse haemorrhage, I had no alternative but to prise open the rigid bone edges and attempt to gain access to the bleeding beneath, forcing a small retractor through the bony incision and cranking it open. But there was no gap between the underside of the bone and heart muscle. The cavernous, thin-walled right ventricle had been plastered by inflammatory adhesions to the bone by a previous wound infection. So I found myself ripping the heart asunder and staring at the underside of the tricuspid valve. Both the hand-held suckers, then the heart itself filled with air as I fought for better access. I then found that this tissue-friendly saw had also transected the right coronary artery. My paralysed registrar simply gaped, as if to say, 'How the fuck are you going to get out of this mess?'

There was nothing I could do in time to save him. Deprived of oxygen, the heart soon fibrillated, so at best – had I persisted – he would have suffered devastating brain injury. So I called time on the gruesome spectacle. The whole shambles had taken less than ten minutes. Apologising to the nurses who had to lay him out and clean the floor, I tossed away my gloves and mask in disgust. The whole bloody catastrophe was straight out of *Saw II* or *Driller Killer*. It felt as if I had driven a bayonet into the man's heart and twisted the blade. Then, just as had been done to me during my formative years, I dispatched the registrar to talk to the man's wife while I went off to the pub.

I didn't see the poor lady again until the inquest, where she sat unaccompanied, listening intently. She bore no malice, nor was the coroner critical in any way. The gruesome fact was that I had unintentionally sawn open that heart and emptied the circulation onto my clogs. In my own mind, I knew that a CT scan would have prompted me to cannulate the man's leg vessels myself, which could have averted the tragedy and was something that I always did after that. Undeterred, I reopened a sternum for the fifth time in front of television cameras just weeks later.

Most deaths in surgery are wholly impersonal. The patient is either covered in drapes on the operating table or obscured by the grim paraphernalia of the intensive care unit. As a result, my most haunting experiences of death stemmed from trauma cases. The sudden, unexpected process of injury pitches an unsuspecting individual into their own Dante's Inferno. Knife and bullet injuries were predictable and easy for me. Cut open the chest, find the haemorrhage, sew up the bleeding points, then refill the circulation with blood – such cases always provoked an adrenaline rush, but usually involved young, healthy tissues to repair.

My own worst nightmare wasn't caused by a gun or a knife. As a young consultant I was once fast-bleeped to the emergency department to help with an incoming road accident. It was still what was called the 'swoop, scoop and run' era, so the patient was being brought in directly without transfusion of cold fluid to screw up the blood clotting. With foresight and sensitivity, the police had already warned reception what to expect, but unfortunately I'd not been party to that. I was outside in the ambulance bays enjoying the sunshine when the vehicle came thundering up the drive, siren blaring and blue lights flashing. When the rear doors were thrown open, the crew wanted a doctor to take a look before they risked moving the patient again.

I could hear the whimpering before I could see the girl, but I knew from the paramedic's grim expression that it was something unpleasant. Unusually awful, in fact. The teenage motorcyclist was lying on her left side, covered by a blood-soaked white sheet. This sheet and what I could see of her face were the same colour. The poor girl had been drained of blood. Normally she would have been shunted quickly through to the resuscitation room, but there was every reason not to rush.

The paramedics quietly and deliberately drew back the sheet so I could see that the girl was transfixed by a fence post. A witness had watched her motorcycle swerve to avoid a deer, then she veered off the road, smashing through a fence into a field. She was left skewered like meat on a kebab stick. The fire brigade eventually released her by sawing through the fence and lifting her free. This left the stake protruding from her blood-soaked blouse. The response of the gathering team was to glare incongruously at the gruesome transfixion and ignore that horrified face behind the oxygen mask.

I took her cold, clammy hand more in clinical assessment than humanity. She was in circulatory shock, not to mention profound mental turmoil. Her pulse rate was around 120 beats per minute, but the fact that I could feel it suggested that her blood pressure was still above 50 mm Hg. Before we moved her I needed to scrutinise the anatomical features of the injury so as to predict what damage we would be confronted with. I had seen several cases of transfixion trauma where the patient survived because the implement narrowly missed or pushed aside all the vital organs. Here the degree of shock indicated otherwise. It was time to get some cannulas in place in a calm and controlled manner, and bring group O negative blood ready to transfuse her. And for pity's sake, she deserved a slug of morphine to take the edge off the sheer terror of her predicament.

Some things I knew instinctively. Had the stake damaged the heart or aorta she would have bled out at the scene. Traumatised small arteries will go into spasm, clot and stop the bleeding themselves as long as injudicious clear fluid infusion doesn't raise the blood pressure and blow the clots off. So I surmised that most of the bleeding must be coming from the veins, which do not constrict. I asked the nurses for some scissors to remove her clothing, now stiff with dried blood. It was like cutting through cardboard and opening a window on the grim reality of her situation.

Her pleading brown eyes remained firmly fixated on the stake. I could make out the jagged ends of ribs protruding through macerated fat and pale, bruised skin. The post had entered directly below her right breast, marginally to the right of the midline, and emerged from her body higher up in her back, suggesting that she had slid feet first after tumbling from her motorcycle. My three-dimensional anatomical knowledge left me in no doubt which structures had been damaged. The post must have taken out her diaphragm and liver, the lower lobe of her right lung and probably the largest vein in the body, the inferior vena cava. The lung wasn't a problem. But if her liver was pulped and the veins torn off the cava, I knew that we couldn't fix her. Scrutiny of the post protruding from her back confirmed my fears – there were fragments of both liver and lung on the wooden shards. Everyone knows what liver looks like from the butcher's, while youthful lung is pink and spongy. I recognised both, and it made me sad.

In just seconds on a Saturday morning she had gone from vivacious carefree student to dying swan transfixed like a vampire. With every agonising breath, blood slopped from the wound edges. Whatever the way forward, I had to talk to her. I edged around the trolley and knelt by her head to distract her as the emergency doctors painfully probed with needles to locate an empty vein. With blood and froth dripping from her mouth, she was finding it difficult to breathe, let alone speak. We needed to put her to sleep right there in the ambulance, then get a tube into her windpipe – a seemingly impossible task in that awkward position. By now I was pretty sure that whatever we did she would die. If not soon, it would be in days or weeks as a result of infection and organ failure in the intensive care unit. So whatever else we attempted to do for her, we had to be kind. Do as little as possible to add to her pain.

Staring directly into her eyes I asked her name. I was simply trying to inject a semblance of humanity into the proceedings and relieve the brutality of it all. Stuttering between breaths, she told me she was a law student, like my own daughter Gemma, which added to my discomfort. I took her icy cold fingers in my right hand and rested my left hand on her hair, hoping to obscure that stake from her gaze.

With tears streaming down her cheeks she murmured, 'I'm going to die, aren't I?'

At that point I ceased being the surgeon because I knew she was right. For her last agonising moments on earth I could only comfort her. So I would be her substitute dad for that time. I held her head and told her what she wanted to hear. That we would put her to sleep now and when she awoke everything would be back in its place. The stake would be gone. The pain and fear would be gone. Her shoulders dropped and she felt less tense.

The gadget clipped onto her index finger showed very low oxygen saturation, so we had to move her to give the anaesthetist his chance with the endotracheal tube. Only then could we begin a token effort at resuscitation. I extended my hand to feel her belly, which was distended and tense. As we explained the need to move her, I could sense her consciousness fading.

She whispered, 'Can you tell mum and dad that I love them, and I'm sorry? They never did want me to have that bike.'

Then she coughed up a plug of blood clot. As she rolled backwards the stake shifted, grating audibly against her shattered ribs. Her eyes rolled towards heaven and she slipped away. Whatever blood she had left in her circulation was pouring out over me. But I didn't mind. It was a privilege to be there with her. The junior doctors from the resuscitation room stirred, intending to begin cardiac massage. Without hesitation I told them to back off. What the fuck did they expect to achieve?

The back of the ambulance fell silent with the horror of it all. I would have loved to have dragged that hideous fence post out of her chest – that had to be left to the pathologists. I couldn't bring myself to watch her autopsy, but it confirmed that her diaphragm had been torn away and her pulped liver avulsed from the inferior vena cava.

That balmy summer's evening I went walking through the bluebell woods of Bladon Heath with Monty, my jet black flat-coated retriever. While he chased rabbits, I sat on a fallen tree carpeted in moss and wondered if there was a God. Where was he on those fraught occasions when I needed some divine intervention? Where was he today when that poor girl tried to avoid hurting a deer and was killed by her kindness? I visualised her devastated parents sitting with a cold corpse in the mortuary, holding their daughter as I'd done in the ambulance, beseeching God to turn the clock back.

There was no point trying to be logical about religion. I knew that high-ranking Oxford – and indeed Cambridge – academics scoffed at the deity concept. Both Richard Dawkins and Stephen Hawking had that gold-plated atheistic confidence in their own abilities, spurning outside help. I guess I was the same. But I would still sneak into the back of a college auditorium and listen to debates on the subject. Some disputed God's existence because of all the evil and misery in the world, and while I could identify with that, I had contrary and privileged insight through the odd patient who actually claimed to have reached the Pearly Gates before we clawed them back.

These vivid out-of-body experiences were rare but occasionally compelling. One spiritual lady described floating calmly on the ceiling as she watched me pumping her heart with my fist through an open chest. Forty minutes into this internal cardiac massage my thumb tore through into her right ventricle – she clearly recalled my words: 'Oh shit, we've had it now.' Fortunately, the perfusionists arrived with the circulatory support system I needed to keep her alive, and I succeeded in repairing the hole.

She uncannily related her memory of the events a number of weeks later in the clinic. Having been party to her own resuscitation attempts from above, she had floated through the clouds to meet with St Peter. This journey amid peace and tranquillity contrasted sharply with our gruesome efforts back down on the ground. But having arrived in heaven she was told she had to return to earth and wait her turn again – a ridiculously close-run thing between me and Grim Reaper. Perhaps God changed as he got older. Maybe he started out with the best of intentions but became cynical and less caring with time. Just like the NHS.

It was only after retiring from surgery that I began to reflect on my role in dispatching so many to that great hospital in the sky. One tranquil spot on the heath still holds a great deal of significance for me. It is a haunted place, a gap in the woodland that overlooks both Blenheim Palace, where my hero Winston Churchill was born, and St Martin's Church, Bladon, where he is buried. A few yards from this clearing a jet plane that had just taken off from Oxford Airport crashed and exploded.

My son Mark was working for exams in his bedroom and watched the whole spectacle unfold. Heroically, he was the first to reach the drama in the field but could do nothing amid the conflagration. He watched the cockpit burn and cremate the occupants. Obviously at seventeen he had a different constitution to his lobotomised father, so the dismal spectacle disturbed him as it might any normal person. As a result he needed medication for post-traumatic stress, which scrambled his memory and cognition at that critical time. After dropping a single grade in biology he was dumped by his chosen university. I was very bitter about that. I still am.

One day when we reached this sacred ground, Monty spotted a stag silhouetted against the evening sky a hundred or so yards up the ride. A shaft of evening sunlight shone through the trees to illuminate a clump of fading bluebells, their heads dipping at the end of their season. Was that majestic stag in fact God looking down on me, surrounded by the spirits I had set free during my career, the ghosts of operations past?

In truth, I had always been a loner. I was still a restless insomniac who would wake in the early hours and write, making stupid notes on material I would never use, continuing to invent impossible operations that no one would ever perform. Did I miss surgery? Not at all, surprisingly enough. Forty years had been plenty. But it remained a great mystery to me how I had achieved so much from my humble beginnings in the backstreets of a northern steel town. Perhaps it was that battle to escape obscurity that provided the momentum. I wanted to be different, and I had the ruthless ambition to take on the system and overcome my past.

Although I spent my whole career writing textbooks and scientific papers for the profession, I reflected for many years on whether it was appropriate to discuss my battles in a public forum. Ironically it was my own patients who urged me to do so, even the loved ones of some who died. So many were eager for their stories to be told. From my own perspective, I always found the history of modern heart surgery to be among the most compelling stories ever told. As a trainee in London and the US I actually knew a number of the pioneers personally, and they had shared their own trials and tribulations with me face to face, encouraging me to make a difference, not to sit in the shadows avoiding conflict. And I certainly attracted trouble right from the start.

The government's policy of releasing named-surgeon death rates to the press was another factor that edged me towards writing a tome for consumption by the general public. What is life really like on the other side of the fence? Is it different from being a statistician, politician or a journalist? The barrister and medical ethicist Daniel Sokol wrote in the *British Medical Journal*, 'The public has an appetite for glimpses of the private lives and thoughts of doctors. They demystify a profession that was once deemed blessed with magical powers.' Perhaps some of us still do have mystical powers. There are few things more intriguing than delivering electricity into a patient's head through a metal plug screwed into their skull like Dr Frankenstein's monster or reinventing human circulation with continuous blood flow without a pulse. These innovations may be construed as witchcraft, but they were my own practical solutions to the terrible illness that is heart failure. Sokol went on to say that doctors are in the habit of revealing 'not the chiselled frame of Apollo … but the wart covered body of Mr Burns, the *Simpsons* character'. But Burns was the rich factory owner. I'm more of a sensitive intellectual, like Bart Simpson's father Homer.

As is often the case, the French have a phrase for it: 'se mettre à nu', to get naked. So that is what I decided to do, although this was a much more interesting spectacle in my younger years than now. My own insight tells me that the public are happier to learn that their surgeon, even a heart or brain surgeon, is human and subject to the same core emotions as anyone else. But because of a freak sporting accident, some qualities possessed by the vast majority of people were lost to me for a while, which proved an unexpected but substantial boost to a career at the sharp end – life perpetually on the 'knife's edge'.

1

family

WHEN I SEARCHED THE INTERNET for a contemporary description of the surgical personality, I found this:

> Testosterone-infused swagger, confident, brash, charismatic, commanding. Arrogant, volatile, even bullying and abusive. Aggressive. Cuts first, asks questions later, because to cut is to cure and the best cure is cold steel. Sometimes wrong but never in doubt. Good with his hands but no time to explain. Compassion and communication are for sissies.

The psychologist author argued that the highly stressful, adrenaline-fuelled environment in which surgeons work attracts a certain personality type. And so it does. Cutting into people, then wallowing in blood, bile, shit, pus or bone dust is such an alien pastime for normal folk that the mere process of operating immediately sets us apart. Those with introspection and self-doubt select themselves out from my specialty.

It is hard to describe how agonisingly difficult it was to gain access to a cardiac surgery training programme in the 1970s, when open heart surgery with the heart–lung machine was only in its second decade. The surgeons of that era were an unashamedly elitist group with the guts, skill and sheer daring to expose a sick heart and attempt to repair it. Methods to protect the muscle when it was starved of blood were frequently inadequate, and prolonged interaction between blood and the foreign surfaces of the bypass machine triggered a damaging inflammatory reaction known as the 'post-perfusion syndrome'. Heart surgeons therefore needed above all to work against the clock – deaths were a daily occurrence, yet most patients were so sick that this wasn't considered a catastrophe. While survival and symptomatic relief were gratifying, death put an end to suffering. Consequently, most families were grateful that their loved ones had at least a chance of their condition improving through surgical intervention.

We all had to go through general surgery training first to show that we had what it takes. First, good hands – and you have to be born that way. Most organs just sit there while you cut and sew them, but the heart is a moving target, a bag of blood under pressure that bleeds torrentially if you bugger it up. Just touching it clumsily can provoke disorganised rhythm and sudden cardiac arrest. Second, the right temperament – the ability to explain death to grieving relatives and to bounce back from a bollocking in the operating theatre. Then courage – the bravery to take over from the boss when he's had enough, the guts to take responsibility for the post-operative care of tiny babies or to address a catastrophe in the trauma room when the nearest consultant is an hour away. Then patience and resilience – being able to stand there as first assistant for six hours without losing concentration, sometimes with a hangover, or to face five days continuously on call in the hospital, day and night without respite. That was surgical training in those days.

A series of infernal exams to become a fellow of the Royal College of Surgeons was an additional burden over and above the clinical work. These covered every aspect of surgery and only a third of the candidates passed each time. It didn't matter that I wanted to operate in the chest. For the 'primary' fellowship we were required to know the anatomy of a human being in minute detail, brain to asshole, teeth to tits – every nerve, artery and vein in the whole body, where they went, what they did, what happened if we damaged them. We had to learn the physiological processes of every organ and the biochemistry of every cell. After some basic operative experience, the 'final' fellowship examined us on the pathology of every surgical condition in the book, then the diagnostic and surgical techniques for each specialty. Only after conclusively demonstrating comprehensive knowledge and skills were we allowed to move on and specialise. I failed both the primary and final fellowship on first sitting, an expensive exercise. Most of my associates did too. The whole miserable process was there to sort the wheat from the chaff, and I wasn't fazed by failure. It was just like rugby, the sport I loved above all others. Some games you won, others you lost.

The surgical world resembles the army. The consultants are the officers and the gentlemen, the trainees line up in tiers through the ranks: senior house officer is equivalent to corporal, registrar acting as sergeant, senior registrar akin to a non-commissioned officer doing all the work and eventually being promoted to the officer's mess. That final step was the most competitive of all. For the ruthlessly ambitious it had to be a top teaching hospital. Heart surgeons strove for London hospitals like the Royal Brompton, the Hammersmith, Guy's or St Thomas'. Appointment to one of these, and you had made it big time. In those days Cambridge had a vibrant cardiothoracic centre in Papworth village out of town. Oxford was doing very little.

All this took place during our formative years, our late twenties and early thirties, when normal people cement relationships, settle down in one location and start a family. Trainee surgeons lived like gypsies, moving from city to city – wherever the best posts were advertised. Something about being a surgeon elevated us to a different plane. We were the fighting cocks of the doctors' mess, the flash Harrys who constantly strove to outdo each other and ruthlessly coveted the top jobs; the guys – and at that time, as now, it was almost exclusively guys – who stayed in the hospital night after night seeking every chance to operate, or, if it was quiet, drifting across to the nurses' quarters, where other exciting action was easy to find.

I was a backstreet kid from Scunthorpe who had married his childhood sweetheart from the local grammar school. Caught up in this whirlwind of ruthless ambition, things changed and marriage became an unintended casualty. I was ashamed of this, but I knew some surgical teams where every member, from junior houseman to consultant, was having an affair in the hospital. Grim in reality, but the stuff of television soaps that glamorise adultery. So widespread was the problem that the Johns Hopkins Hospital in Baltimore carried out a formal study of divorce as an occupational hazard in medicine. The younger their residents were when they married, the higher their divorce rate. Understandably, divorce was commonplace when the spouse did not work in the medical field. Blame it on the communication gap. They had little to talk about because doctors – and especially surgeons – are engrossed in their hospital life.

The Johns Hopkins study showed that more than half of psychiatrists and one in three surgeons divorced. Cardiac surgery had an impressive divorce rate, which I already knew from my colleagues' experience. Reasons cited were high testosterone levels, long hours and nights in the hospital, and close working relationships with numerous attractive young women, often in stressful and emotional circumstances. Professional bonds are formed, and these evolve into romance. At one stage the Dean of Duke University Medical School saw fit to warn applicants that the institution was experiencing a greater than 100 per cent divorce rate. Why exceeding the maximum? Because students showed up already married, got divorced, then remarried and divorced a second time. They all lived a life in which work was seen to come first, with everything else a distant second.

Once at a conference in California I picked up a copy of *Pacific Standard* magazine that contained an article entitled 'Why are so many surgeons assholes?'. Obviously it was about prevailing personality types. A scrub nurse friend of the journalist described an incident in the operating theatre where she had passed the sharp scalpel to the surgeon and he lacerated his thumb on the blade. Now furious, he shouted at her, 'What kind of pass was that. What are we, two kids in the playground with Play-Doh? Ridiculous.' Then to emphasise his point he threw the scalpel back at her. The nurse was horrified, but as she didn't know how to react she just kept quiet. No one stood up for her, and no one ever reprimanded the surgeon for being aggressive or throwing the sharp instrument. The inference was that this is how a lot of surgeons behaved and they get away with it all the time.

I have known many surgeons who threw instruments around the room, and although I never aimed one at an assistant I did use to toss faulty instruments onto the floor. It meant that I couldn't be given them a second time. Having said that, most successful surgeons have certain malign traits in common. These have been summarised in the medical literature as the 'dark triad' of psychopathy, Machiavellianism – the callous attitude in which the ends are held to justify the means – and narcissism, which manifests as the excessive self-absorption and sense of superiority that goes with egoism and an extreme need for attention from others. This dark triad emanates from placing personal goals and self-interest above the needs of other people.

Just in the last few months psychologists at the University of Copenhagen have shown that if a person manifests just one of these dark personality traits, they probably have them all simmering below the surface, including so-called moral disengagement and entitlement, which enables someone to throw surgical instruments with absolutely no conscience at all. This detailed mapping of the dark triad is comparable to Charles Spearman's demonstration a hundred years ago that people who score highly in one type of intelligence test are likely to perform equally well in other kinds. Perhaps the daunting road to a surgical career inadvertently selects characters with these negative traits. It certainly appears that way, yet I had a very different side to my personality when it came to my own family. Maritally I fell into the same old traps, but I would go to any lengths to make my children happy or my parents proud.

I was not rostered to be in surgery as it was my daughter Gemma's birthday and I hoped to be free. The phantom father who had let her down so many times in the past, I planned to drive to Cambridge in the afternoon to surprise her. Then I discovered that three of our five surgeons were out of town. Two were committed to outreach clinics at district hospitals trying to bring in 'customers', as the NHS now called them, or better still the odd private patient. The third was away at a conference, one of those

academically destitute commercial meetings at a glamor-
ous resort paid for by the sponsor, with business-class
flights and all the rest. As a gullible young consultant I
had enjoyed these trips, but it eventually wears thin – tedious airports, buckets of alcohol and forced comradery
with competitive colleagues who would cheerfully drive
their scalpel into your back the minute it was all over.

It was this surgeon's operating list that lay vacant, and
the unit manager had twisted my arm to stand in for him.
To let an operating theatre with a full complement of staff
lie idle for the day was a criminal waste of resources, so I
reluctantly agreed to the request. I had built this unit from
nothing to being virtually the largest in the country, not
that anyone could give a shit. The management changed
so frequently that history was soon forgotten, dispatched
to oblivion by the quagmire of financial expediency. So
my daughter would have to wait. Again.

When I asked Sue, my secretary, to find two urgent
waiting-list patients at short notice, I didn't mention the
birthday. Just two cases should see me on the road by
mid-afternoon. I suggested that one should be the infant
girl with Down's syndrome who had been cancelled twice
before. She was in danger of becoming inoperable because
of excessive blood flow and rising pressure in the artery
to the lungs. I bore special affection for these children.
When I started out in cardiac surgery, many considered it
inappropriate to repair their heart defects. I couldn't get
my head around a policy that discriminated against kids
with a particular condition, so ultimately I overcompen-
sated by taking them on as desperately debilitated young

adults – trying to turn the clock back, sometimes without success.

The second case needed to be more straightforward. Sue had repeatedly been pestered by a self-styled VIP who held some snooty position in a neighbouring health authority. When I reviewed this lady in the outpatient clinic, she took exception to my suggesting that weight loss would not only improve her breathlessness but reduce the risks during her mitral valve surgery. I was sternly reminded that she had featured in a recent honours list, presumably for services dedicated to getting her onto an honours list, as is frequently the case in healthcare. I wasn't in the slightest bit impressed – and she could see that. But she kept insisting on an early date and I couldn't blame Sue for wanting her out of the way. The titled lady wouldn't make first slot on the list, however. That was for the baby. A third cancellation was not an option.

6 am. As I set out for work from Woodstock, my home in Oxfordshire, shafts of sunlight burst through the turrets of Blenheim Palace like rays of optimism. I would be seeing Gemma on her birthday. When she was born I was nowhere to be found, and I'd spent twenty years trying to make up for that. Sue, who also suffers from traffic phobia, joined me in the office before 7 am, and we soon dispensed with the paperwork that I had to do before the adult intensive care ward round at 7.30. The day's operating lists were already displayed on a white board at the main nurse's station. The male charge nurse knew that my only adult patient was unlikely to reach the unit until mid-afternoon, but still felt obliged to warn me that beds

were tight. Glancing towards the row of empty beds surrounded by unplugged ventilators and cardiac monitors, I didn't need to ask. It was more of the same. 'Tight on beds' means not enough nurses. In the NHS, every intensive care bed must have a dedicated nurse. In other countries they double up quite safely to get the work done, but here we just cancel operations as if they were appointments with the hairdresser.

On this particular morning I didn't know many of the nurses' faces – and they didn't recognise me. This told me that the night shift had relied heavily on agency staff. Two of my three cases from the previous day could leave the unit, but only when ward beds became available. Until then, they would continue to languish in this intimidating environment that never slept, at a cost exceeding £1,000 per day. Sometimes we'd even discharge patients directly home from intensive care when the ward was chronically blocked with the elderly and the destitute.

This was not how it used to be. When we fought to build the department, just three heart surgeons would perform 1,500 heart operations each year and we'd cover the chest surgery between us. Now in the same modest facilities we had five heart surgeons performing half that number of cases, alongside another three chest surgeons operating on the lungs. This was the price of progress – twice as many highly trained professionals doing much less work amid a disintegrating infrastructure. But hey. A hospital delegation was trying to recruit nurses in the Philippines that very week, so all would be well one day.

8 am – and my early-morning optimism was already punctured. I left the cacophony of life support, pulsating balloon pumps, hissing ventilators and screeching alarms. I heard weeping relatives, suggesting that a bed might soon be vacated. Knife to skin should be at 8.30, and I expected the baby to be anaesthetised by now. I assiduously avoided watching parents part from their children at the operating theatre doors. It was traumatic enough for me when my son had his tonsils out. Heart operations were a cut above. When I told parents that their child had a 95 per cent chance of survival, all that registered was the 5 per cent possibility of death. Statistics don't help when it's your child that doesn't make it. So I told them what they wanted to hear, then hoped it would be true.

But the anaesthetic room was empty. The anaesthetist was sitting in the coffee room eating breakfast.

'Have we sent yet?' I asked with an air of resignation.

She shook her head. We had to wait for the paediatric intensive care ward round to decide whether they could give us a bed. No bed, third cancellation. It couldn't be allowed to happen, yet the round hadn't even started. It was an 8.30 start at the other end of the corridor, so I went there directly. With rising blood pressure, I still tried to remain polite. The staff had desperately sick children to care for and my little patient was just another anonymous name in the diary, followed by the words 'atrioventricular canal'. The whole centre of her heart was missing and her lungs were flooded. With every day that passed, her chances of survival decreased.

The trouble was that I loved the children's intensive care unit. That little enclave of rooms was my escape from the rest of the hospital, a place that always put life – and my own troubles – in perspective. Only special people could survive the heartache in that place. The nurses liked to work with my heart surgery cases because the vast majority got better, a welcome relief from the ravages of children's cancer, septicaemia or road-traffic accidents that they also had to deal with. The worst things in the world happened there, but everyone came back the next day to start all over again.

Every one of the cots had a little body in it, with fretful family groups gathered around. My eyes fixed on a pair of gangrenous arms – the meningococcal meningitis child I'd watched for weeks, hanging on to life. The mother knew me well enough by now, seeing my babies come and go with happy parents. I always asked her how things were going, she always smiled. Today they were going to amputate those black, mummified limbs. No more little hands or tiny fingers. They would just drop off, with a little help to tidy things up.

I asked whether there was any chance of a bed by lunchtime, so that we could at least send for the baby. Sister really didn't want to let me down. One of her day-shift nurses was already in the radiology department with a head-trauma victim who'd been hit by a speeding car on the way to school. Should the injuries prove as severe as feared, ventilatory support would be withdrawn. Then my case could go to theatre. I enquired whether the organ donor phrase had been mentioned.

'Do you want the bed or don't you?' she replied. 'That route could take us well into tomorrow.'

For comfort I picked up a bacon sandwich, then wandered off in my theatre gear through the hordes who arrived for work at nine o'clock. These were normal people who didn't have to split breast-bones, stop hearts or give desolate parents bad news, such as 'Your child's operation is cancelled again.' Now the dilemma. Should I give up on the little girl, then send for the VIP and her mitral repair? The lady wouldn't have been starved long enough or had a pre-med, but at least I could take off to Cambridge to see my daughter afterwards without the worry of leaving a newly operated infant when I wasn't on call. Or should I hold out for the possibility of a bed for her parents' sake?

Turning away from blank faces and the tacit acceptance of dysfunctionality, I diverted to radiology. They knew me well enough at the CT scanner and seemed relieved to discover that I was not attempting to take over their next slot. The images of the child's battered brain emerged slice by slice. The skull had been cracked open like the top of a boiled egg. Where there should have been clear lakes of cerebrospinal fluid, there was nothing. The brain surgeon and intensive care doctors shook their heads in dismay. Nothing would be gained by operating. The cerebral cortex was pulp and the brain stem had herniated through the base of the skull. I was relieved that I couldn't see that poor broken body concealed within the scanner. She had toddled off happily to the village school; now she hovered between earth and heaven, her brain already gone. So I had my intensive care bed. Relief for one set of parents, complete and utter desolation for another.

Striding purposefully back to the operating theatres, I requested that they send directly for my first case. The agency anaesthetic nurse hadn't the faintest idea who I was and confronted me with the usual crap, saying that they hadn't heard if there was a bed yet.

Uncharacteristically, and because I didn't know the woman, I lost the plot and shouted, 'I'm telling you there's a fucking bed. Now send for the child.'

The anaesthetist stood in the doorway and gave me a long, hard stare. The nurse picked up the phone and called the paediatric intensive care unit sister. At that moment, I worried that others had not been informed that the trauma case was not for ventilation. But I got lucky. The response confirmed my outburst. Yes, we could send for the cardiac case.

To put the baby asleep and insert cannulas into her tiny blood vessels would take an hour, so to avoid the transmitted anxiety from the parents' tearful separation from their baby girl, I slipped into the anaesthetic room of the thoracic theatre, carrying a plastic cup of ghastly grey coffee. This time I was warmly greeted by an old friend, whom I asked to measure my blood pressure. It was 180/100 – far too high, despite the daily blood pressure medication I had been taking for ten years.

As the fearful parents shuffled past the door I heard one of them say, 'Please tell Professor Westaby we are grateful for this chance.' I suspected they still didn't believe that their baby would make it. Perhaps they were worried that we wouldn't try as hard as we could because of the Down's syndrome.

Would a concert pianist prepare for an important recital by first enduring three hours of intense frustration? Would a watchmaker have to face a blazing row before assembling a complicated Rolex movement? My job was to reconfigure a deformed heart the size of a walnut, yet I enjoyed zero consideration for my state of mind from those around me. I wouldn't so much as get on a bus if the driver was subject to that much irritation. The first time I stood as the operating surgeon looking into the void at the centre of an atrioventricular canal defect, I thought, 'Shit, what the hell do I do with this?' Yet I always succeeded in separating the left and right sides of the heart with patches, then creating new mitral and tricuspid valves from the rudimentary valve tissue. It's complex work, but I never lost one on the operating table.

I finally ran the stainless-steel blade through the baby's skin at 11 am. As the first drops of blood skidded over the plastic drape, I remembered that I had not made contact with my daughter. That thought hit me just as the oscillating saw bisected the baby's sternum, but there was nothing I could do about it now. I needed complete focus to reconfigure that tiny deformed heart and give the baby a lifetime without breathlessness or pain. So what did I need to consider? The new mitral valve must not leak, although it wouldn't be too bad if there was a whiff of regurgitation through the tricuspid valve on the low-pressure side of the circulation. And we had to be careful not to damage the invisible electrical conduction system that crucially coordinates the heart's contraction and relaxation. Otherwise she would need a permanent pacemaker. At that point I felt it would have been much easier to be a watchmaker or concert pianist ...

As it turned out, that little heart would be the least of my problems that day. I separated the chambers with obsessively sewn patches of Dacron cloth, then carefully created the new valves upon which the baby's future depended. It was much the same as operating within an egg cup. When blood was reintroduced into the tiny coronary arteries the little heart took off like an express train. Just as I prepared to separate the baby from the heart–lung machine, a pale and worried face appeared at the theatre door.

'Sorry, Professor,' the woman said, 'but we need you right now in Theatre 2. Mr Maynard is in trouble.'

'How much trouble?' I asked, without diverting my eyes from the baby's heart.

'The patient is bleeding from a hole in the aorta and he can't stop it.' She had a note of desperation in her voice.

Although the baby seemed fine, I would not normally leave a registrar to remove the bypass cannulas and close up. But it needed a snap decision. On the balance of probabilities, I decided that I should try to help. In haste, I forgot that I was tethered by the electric cable of my powerful head lamp. Standing back from the operating table, I avulsed the bloody thing. Several hundred pounds' worth of damage in two seconds.

Nick Maynard was a first-rate upper gastrointestinal surgeon who specialised in stomach and oesophageal cancer. He dealt with tubes normally filled with food and air, not blood at high pressure. But this unfortunate patient did not have cancer. Just days before, she had been completely well. While happily eating sea bass in a fancy restaurant she swallowed a fish bone. At first the discomfort abated and she could swallow. Then a dull ache emerged deep in the chest, next a swinging fever with night sweats. Soon just swallowing liquids became difficult and made the pain worse. The GP knew she was in trouble. Blood results sent from the surgery showed a very high white blood cell count, which suggested an abscess. Rather than passing through the gut as most bones do, this one had clearly penetrated through the wall of the oesophagus.

Nick's team was surrounded by medical students and radiologists as the CT scans came through. There was an abscess the size of an orange wedged between oesophagus and aorta in the back of her chest. Worryingly, there were bubbles of gas in the pus. Gas-forming organisms are among the most dangerous, so it was no surprise that she felt dreadful. The pus needed to be drained away urgently before the bugs entered her blood stream and caused septicaemia. Otherwise it could be fit to fatal within days.

The oesophagus and aorta descend side by side in the chest, nestled behind the heart and in front of the spine – oesophagus on the right, aorta to the left. Tiger country. Under high-dose antibiotic cover, Nick planned to open the right side of the chest through the ribs and locate the abscess behind the lung. Then, by opening the abscess cavity, the pus could be washed out and drains left in place for a few days until the antibiotics clobbered the infection. Nick thought that the small perforation through the muscular wall of the oesophagus would seal itself. While awfully simple in theory, it was destined to be simply awful.

Through the glass door of Theatre 2, I could see Nick, sweating profusely with his face covered in blood, and both arms up to the elbows in the woman's chest. Blood was slopping out of the chest cavity and down his blue gown, while anaesthetists were squeezing in bags of blood. It transpired that all had gone according to plan until he swept an index finger around the abscess cavity to clear the infected debris. First came the noxious odour of anaerobic bacteria and rotting flesh. Then, whoosh! Blood hit the operating lights. The abscess had eroded through the wall of the aorta. Behind the heart lay an infected swamp. All Nick could do was to stick his fist into the fountain and press hard. Big problem. They had already lost more than a litre of blood and if his fist moved she would bleed out in seconds.

Groaning deeply under the burden of the day, I gave Nick a resigned look and thought for a moment. The bleeding was still not under control and there was no prospect of repairing the hole while her heart kept on pumping. She would simply bleed to death. The only potential route out of the predicament – I called it 'deep shit' at the time – was to get onto cardiopulmonary bypass, cool her down to 16°C, then stop the circulation altogether. Deep cooling of the brain would give us a safe thirty- to forty-minute window without blood flow to identify and deal with the damage.

Given the morning's conflict, I very politely asked anyone not immediately engaged in the frantic resuscitation to ask one of my perfusionists to bring in and prepare a heart–lung machine. And for a couple of my own scrub nurses and a specialist cardiac anaesthetist to come across. Nick just had to keep on pressing. His anaesthetists kept on squeezing.

Once I'd scrubbed up and joined the team around the body, I couldn't even see the heart. I needed a much bigger hole in the chest to work around my colleague's 'finger in the dyke'. There was no time for finesse. With the scalpel and cautery I virtually split her in half as she lay there, right side uppermost on the operating table. The metal retractor cranked the chest wide apart with a crack that told me that one of her ribs had just broken. This was not unusual. Chest surgery is a brutal business.

Now I could see the pale, empty heart beating rapidly in its fibrous sac. I needed to cut this open and insert two cannulas to connect to the bypass machine. The first went into the aorta as it left the left ventricle carrying cherry-red oxygenated blood. The second was pushed into the empty right atrium, where blue blood from the veins of the body re-entered the heart to be pumped to the lungs. This venous blood, low in oxygen, would now pass through a heat exchanger and mechanical oxygenator before re-entering the aorta. Then we could cool and protect the brain and other vital organs. The heart is rarely approached through the right chest, but I had done it on a number of occasions for complex reoperations on the mitral valve. With a daunting challenge like this, every ounce of experience counted.

Thinking ahead, I told one of the watching cardiac registrars to go in person to the homograft bank and ask for a tube of antibiotic-treated aorta from the supply of spare parts we obtained from dead donors at autopsy with the relatives' permission. Human tissue is more resistant to infection than synthetic vascular grafts made from Dacron fabric. I often used donated heart valves, patches of aorta or segments of blood vessels from the dead to repair the living. This is recycling. God's stuff is still better than man-made.

At 2 pm the registrar from Theatre 5 came in to announce that he had put in pacemaker wires and chest drains, and had closed the baby's chest. All was well.

It took us around thirty minutes to cool down for the next stage of the operation. While his hands grew colder and colder, I congratulated Nick for saving the woman's life. I told him not to risk moving and that cold was good as it meant the woman's brain was cooling too. Then I asked the enthusiastic registrar to scrub up and babysit the bypass circuit so I could duck out for coffee and a piss. What I really wanted to do was to phone Gemma, but when I did there was no answer. She was still in a seminar. Although time was passing relentlessly, I remained hopeful that I would be in Cambridge by the evening.

At 18°C I was too impatient to wait any longer. Gowned and gloved for the third time that day, I told the perfusionist to stop the pump and empty the lady's circulation into the blood reservoir. Nick could finally withdraw his cold, stiff arms from her chest after having had them in there for more than an hour, while I took the first operator's position. In turn, Nick moved the registrar out of the way, eager to get a look at the damage for himself.

With no blood flowing around the body, we were working against the clock. The infected tissues had the consistency of wet blotting paper and the stench of rotten cabbage. We could not repair the damaged oesophagus, and Nick agreed it had to go. I chopped through the precious muscular tube above and below the abscess, and dissected it away from the aorta. Nick passed a wide-bore suction tube down into the stomach to prevent it from spewing acid and bile over my aortic repair.

Now we had a clear view of the ragged hole, which really should have been a fatal problem. I reluctantly decided to replace the whole infected segment of aorta with the homograft tube rather than risk just a patch. No time to debate this. I trimmed the donor tube to the correct length, then sewed at top speed using blue polyester thread on a fine stainless-steel needle, held in a long titanium needle holder; deep bites into healthy tissue – aesthetically pleasing, bordering on the erotic. Throwing the final knot left-handed, I told Richard the perfusionist to 'go back on' and rewarm. Cold blood from the machine expanded the flaccid graft and air fizzed through the needle holes. It needed a couple of extra stitches to make the whole repair blood tight, but we restored blood flow to the brain after thirty-two minutes. Happy days. Though not so happy in my own case.

I really didn't have time to loiter and admire my needle-work. Between us we agreed that Nick would divert the upper end of the oesophagus out of the left side of the poor lady's neck to drain saliva and enable her to swallow liquids for comfort. The lower end would then be closed off and an entrance to the stomach fashioned through the abdominal wall through which she would now be fed. We call this a gastrostomy. Months down the line Nick would restore her swallowing with a new gullet made by trans-posing a length of large bowel between her neck and stomach. But for now she was safe. In life, and for that matter death, timing is everything. Heart surgeon close at hand. Heart–lung machine and perfusionist available between cases. Spare parts on the shelf. Otherwise she was dead, killed by a fish.

Nick's gastro team were happy to close the chest, put in the drains and finish off. Stepping backwards from the table into a pool of slippery blood clot, I skidded grace-lessly onto my backside, hard down on the tiled floor with a crack – retribution perhaps for leaving Nick for so long with his cold hands in the chest. Now with a soggy red patch on my trousers and the suspense of a near-death drama lifted, it gave the nurses something to laugh at. Some proffered concern for the integrity of my coccyx. But, pain apart, I was content to have dispelled the gloom.

The levity was short-lived as no fewer than four messages with my name attached were taped to the door. First, the lady waiting for the mitral repair on the ward was agitated and wanted to see me. Predictable. Second, would I go to the paediatric intensive care unit where the baby was losing a little too much blood into the drains? Shit. Next, a lady doctor in the accident department of the Norfolk and Norwich Hospital was trying to get hold of me. Why on earth would that be? It was many miles away. And last, the medical director would like to see me in his office with the director of nursing at 4 pm.

Bugger that. It was already 4.10, and I was in no doubt what the chat would be about – swearing at the unhelpful agency nurse, quite inappropriate conduct for a consultant surgeon. Another ticking off. Nor was I in the mood for an acrimonious discussion with the cancelled mitral lady. After 5 pm there were only sufficient nurses to staff one emergency theatre. The nurses would never allow me to begin an elective operation at this time of day. So my only concern was for the baby. Was it significant surgical bleeding or just oozing through compromised blood clotting after being on the bypass machine? Still hoping to leave town, I went directly to the unit to find out.

The afternoon ward round was congregated around the cot. On either side crouched an anxious parent holding a cool, sweaty little hand. Suspended from the drip stand was a tell-tale bag of donor blood dripping briskly through the jugular vein cannula in the baby's neck. Without reading the levels I could see that there was too much blood in the drains. The precious red stuff was dripping in one end and straight out the other. What's more, they had checked the clotting profile and it was virtually normal.

With that one glance my plans for the evening were dashed. Cambridge might as well have been on a different planet. I had to take the baby back to theatre and stop the bloody bleeding. Abject despair turned to anger. I should have closed the chest myself – but then fishbone lady would be dead now. Acrimoniously I rang my so-called 'helper', telling him to lay claim to the emergency operating theatre and that I would push the cot around myself. Five minutes later Mr Putty Fingers called back to say that they couldn't staff an emergency theatre because the chest surgeons were running late with a lung cancer operation. We would have to wait for them to finish. Until then, no room for emergencies, so keep squeezing in the blood. In the meantime, any remaining chance of seeing my daughter on her birthday had gone. More of the same. Useless absentee father ridden with guilt, and made worse by the fact that I had still not made contact. I was a sorry sight with my bloody trousers and sore bum.

There was no point in trying to rush the chest surgeons. They operate slowly through small holes with telescopes and invariably overestimate what they can squeeze in to an operating list. Yet no access for emergency surgery spells trouble. I was now glued to the cot side, with the fretting parents wanting me to stop the bleeding. I deployed that old chestnut: 'It was alright when I left. It can't be bleeding from the heart.'

Sure enough, over the next thirty minutes the bleeding slowed to a trickle. I fantasised that blood clotting had finally sealed the needle holes, which would allow me to escape the hospital without reopening the chest. Except the jugular veins were distending as the blood loss slowed. Perhaps there was too much transfusion. More likely, the chest drains had blocked off and blood was now accumulating under pressure in the closed space within the pericardium so the right atrium couldn't fill properly – what we call cardiac tamponade. Should the blood pressure begin to fall, we would be in real trouble.

The baby's blood pressure drifted down. We couldn't wait any longer for an operating theatre. Now I needed to reopen the chest right there in the cot and scoop out the blood clot. Sister carried the heavy pre-sterilised thoracotomy kit to the cot side and dumped it on a trolley. Still wearing theatre blues, I hastily scrubbed up at the sink while calling for the registrar who had left me in this mess. He had already gone home, so we tried to find the on-call registrar. It was a locum, who was already scrubbed up in the thoracic theatre.

So I got on and did it without help – it was a very small chest, after all – getting the baby prepared, draped and her sternum wide open in less than two minutes. The suction tubing was not connected yet, so I scooped out the clots with my index finger, then packed the pericardial cavity with virginal white swabs. An expanding bright red spot soon showed me the bleeding point, a continuous trickle from the temporary pacing wire site in the muscle of the right ventricle, ostensibly trivial but life-threatening. That's the way with cardiac surgery. It has to be perfect every time or patients die needlessly.

The cardiac rhythm was normal, so I pulled out the wire and stemmed the dribble with a single mattress stitch. Sure enough the drains were blocked. I changed them for clean ones and closed up. The whole process took ten minutes, but it had been a completely avoidable charade. It transpired that the trainee surgeon lacked the confidence to put a stitch into the baby's twitching ventricle, simply hoping that the oozing would stop. He would not make it in this specialty.

7 pm. I was intrigued by that message from Norwich A&E. Were they still waiting to talk to me in the hospital? At first bewildered, I now became uneasy, paranoid even. Norwich was not far from Cambridge. Could Gemma have been out with friends and had an accident? Why did that not occur to me earlier? So I fretfully called her mobile. This time birthday girl answered cheerily and asked whether I was well on my way. The ensuing silence spoke volumes. There was no way I would get to see either of my children that night. Both patients survived, but part of me died. Again.

2

sadness

7.30 PM. I HAD GIVEN A CHILD a new life then pulled off one of surgery's great saves. I should have been floating on air that evening, but I wasn't. Far from it. I was guilt ridden and inconsolable, still drawn to Cambridge when every element of logic insisted that going there would be futile. I needed to take off for Woodstock and drink myself into oblivion. That bloody phone message was still unanswered – but I wasn't on call. Why on earth should I bother now? Because I always did, I guess. There had to be a reason for it. My life was never my own.

'Good evening. Ipswich Hospital. Which department, please?'

'Accident department, please.'

'Sorry, that line is engaged. Can I put you on hold?'

There followed mindless waiting-forever music, tunes that made minutes seem like hours, time more joyfully spent waiting to be castigated by the medical director.

Then the young doctor was found.

'Thank you, Professor. I know you've been in theatre all day. I'm Lucy, the on-call medical SHO. I was hoping that you would accept an emergency that has been with us for some time. An aortic dissection.' (In medicine, people are frequently referred to by their condition rather than their name.) 'He's a GP and had heart surgery a few years ago – an aortic valve replacement at Papworth.'

'Then why aren't Papworth operating on his aortic dissection?'

There followed an embarrassed silence.

'Their surgeon on call said he had another emergency waiting and we should send the doctor somewhere else.'

I was rather nonplussed by this approach as there were several cardiac centres in London that were closer to Ipswich. Aortic dissection is a dire emergency, where the main artery supplying the whole body suffers a sudden tear through the innermost of its three layers. This exposes the middle layer, which usually splits along its entire length under the high pressure, all the way from just above the valve down to the leg arteries. Branches to the vital organs can be sheared off, interrupting their blood supply and causing stroke, dead gut, pulseless legs or failing kidneys. Worse still, the split aorta is likely to rupture at any time, causing sudden death. And the poor chap was a doctor. He deserved better. Anyone deserved better.

I asked his age and current condition. The man was sixty and had complained of sudden severe chest pain, rapidly followed by paralysis of his right side. That meant he had extensive brain injury caused by the carotid artery supplying the left cerebral hemisphere becoming detached. The longer he was left before surgery, the less likely he was to experience any recovery. The patient couldn't speak but sweet, persistent Lucy remained optimistic, saying that he was still awake and could move his left side.

There was one piece of critical information I didn't have, besides his name, that is. What was his blood pressure? Before committing any patient with dissection to an ambulance or helicopter journey, it was vital that the blood pressure was carefully controlled with intravenous anti-hypertensive drugs because a surge in pressure can easily rupture the damaged vessel. So many patients die during or soon after transfer for that very reason.

'180/100. We can't seem to get it down.' An element of panic had now entered her voice.

What that meant was that all the senior staff had buggered off home and left her to it, and she had never seen such a case before. After a day of conflict and castigation I chose my words carefully.

'Oh shit! You must get that down. Get him on nitroprusside.'

I pictured the paper-thin tissue expanding to bursting point while the dissection process extended further throughout the vascular tree. Even with emergency surgery, one in four of these patients died.

Lucy responded that they didn't want to drop the blood pressure too far because he wasn't passing much urine and the CT scan showed that the left kidney had no blood flow. Only surgery could help fix that, so the sooner we got him onto an operating table the better. Should the guts lose their blood supply, little could be done. I asked whether he had abdominal pain or tenderness. Apparently not, so that was a positive.

This terrified patient had been lying paralysed on a hard hospital trolley for hours, surrounded by his family. He knew his own diagnosis and was fully aware that urgent surgery was his only chance of survival. Worse still, he'd had heart surgery before for an abnormal aortic valve, which is often associated with a weakened aortic wall. Reoperations are much more taxing than virgin surgery, so I summarised the situation in my mind. Physician with the highest-risk acute emergency needs reoperation but has an established stroke and one kidney down. His blood pressure is uncontrolled and he is at least two hours away by road. Could they arrange a heli-copter? No, they had already tried. No wonder Papworth weren't interested!

Lucy sensed that I was wavering. Hedging my bets, I told her that I had no idea whether we had any intensive care beds available.

So Lucy played her trump card. 'The family asked that he be sent to you personally. Apparently you were at medical school together. I think he was a friend of yours.'

What was that question I never asked? Something we don't regard as important – the patient's name. Surgeons are less interested in people. We want problems to fix, but I had already had enough problems for one day.

Suddenly the penny dropped. A GP in Suffolk. My own age and with previous heart surgery. He was a jovial rugby prop forward, captain of the 2nd XV at Charing Cross Hospital, my old mate Steve Norton. We met on our first day at medical school in 1966. I was a shy, unassuming backstreet kid, frightened by my own shadow, and no one from my family had ever been to university before. Steve was an ebullient extrovert, full of confidence, destined to become a much-loved GP in rural Suffolk while I underwent metamorphosis into a fearless operating machine. Same profession, worlds apart. How did that happen?

I just said, 'Bugger the beds. Send him across as fast as you can. I appreciate you should be going off duty, Lucy, but someone must come with him to screw that pressure down. And please send the CT scan.'

With no one to delegate to at this time of the evening, I had to make all the arrangements myself. The on-call nursing team had already worked all day and were just finishing a routine lung cancer operation. They were less than delighted by the prospect of a protracted emergency reoperation, one they expected to take all night. With foot down and blue lights flashing, the ambulance ought to be with us by 11 pm. If Steve survived to see Oxford alive, I would wheel him directly to the anaesthetic room.

Now the battle had started. Was there an empty intensive care bed? If not, there would be a bloody row about accepting a patient from outside the region without asking. Who was the on-call anaesthetist? I got lucky with Dave Pigott, a dour South African who helped with my artificial hearts and revelled in a challenge. Then lucky again that Ayrin was the scrub nurse. She was a diminutive, ultra-polite Filipino girl who never complained about anything because she was proud to work for the NHS.

Her invariable response to any expression of gratitude was 'Welcome.' I used to think that this was the only English word she knew. The perfusionists always moaned and groaned when called at night, but they were all ultra-reliable. I just asked switchboard to call in whoever was on the rota and I looked forward to the surprise.

As the sun went down, we waited. I called home and spoke to my long-suffering wife Sarah, who thought I was in Cambridge and was sad for me that I wasn't. I explained that I was waiting to operate on Steve Norton from medical school and wouldn't be home tonight. That concerned her. I wasn't the duty surgeon, and she remembered the heated discussions when I was faced with the prospect of operating on my own father during his heart attack. In the end, my cardiology colleague Oliver spared me the moral issues by curing him with coronary stents.

Sarah asked tentatively whether I should ask the on-call surgeon to do it. How did I feel about operating on a good friend at such high stakes? Cardiac surgeons are rarely introspective and self-effacing. I answered her question with a question: 'If you had an aortic dissection, who would you want to do the surgery?' Response: 'You.' Well then, why are you surprised that Steve's family felt the same?

As she'd sat by the bedside, Steve's wife Hilary knew the situation was dire. What was the anticipated mortality rate for aortic dissection? An international registry from top cardiac centres in Europe and the United States reported 25 per cent. What is the lowest recorded mortality in any series of cases? Six per cent. Who had operated on those cases? A surgeon in Oxford. So who would give Steve the best chance of coming through this catastrophe? I had no reservations whatever about battling to save my mate. As the phrase goes, 'That's what friends are for.'

Sarah's next question was whether I'd eaten anything that day. This took some time to think about. I recalled a bacon sandwich at the crack of dawn. I told her that I'd find a bag of crisps from a vending machine before we launched into the night's work. But food was the least of my concerns at that point. I needed an experienced first assistant, someone who had operated with me on dissections before, not an inexperienced locum brought in to cover a few night shifts. When the shit hits the fan, a coherent team makes a massive difference. Bums on seats is not the same. Amir was not on call, so I picked up the phone and asked him if he was doing anything. One thing he certainly wouldn't be doing was drinking. He was effusive in his willingness to help, honoured to be dragged in at night to help the boss with a complex case. And I knew that he was capable of standing at the table for hours when I needed someone to stem the bleeding then close up. That was a young man's game.

Steve and Hilary were at my wedding to my first wife Jane. Our pack were all young interns at Charing Cross Hospital after graduating, part of the rugby crowd that never took life too seriously. It was Steve who placed the bet that saw me streak naked the length of Pembridge Gardens to Notting Hill Gate tube station during rush hour. And we had both been fished out of the fountains in

Trafalgar Square after a rugby club bash in Fleet Street, only to spend a cold night in Bow Street nick. I failed anatomy that term. Escapades long forgotten, just flashbacks for me as he travelled paralysed and semi-conscious through the night, unexpectedly perched on the edge of life. Once good friends, we were now surgeon and patient, something I never expected nor wanted to happen.

I wandered the silent hospital corridors to pass the time, consciously avoiding a confrontation with cardiac intensive care. I would let Pigott tell them we had an emergency once we were in theatre. Or maybe I'd ask Amir, who joined me in general intensive care, where we visited the fishbone lady. The 'great save', whose name I never knew, was beginning to wake up, her bed surrounded by her anxious daughters, arms extended to their mother's cold hands under the warming blanket. Predictably, she had 'after-cooled' down to 34°C following the hypothermic circulatory arrest and was now shivering violently. Shivering, and the vasoconstriction response to cold, had pushed her blood pressure up to astronomical levels and Amir realised that this was likely to burst the repair.

The lady night registrar nonchalantly strolled across, clearly uncertain about whom she was about to address.

'Can I help you?' she enquired in an aloof manner, presuming that this scruffy visitor in theatre blues was a porter or something. My response must have come as a surprise.

'No, but you can help this lady by getting her blood pressure down before she blows her bloody graft off. Paralyse her and keep her asleep until morning.'

The daughters were wide-eyed. The implications of my reply were lost on them, but they sensed an air of tension between the players.

'Give her a bolus of propranolol right now,' Amir chipped in assertively.

Registrar lady was now defensive and flustered, verging on shocked. She was not much older than my birthday girl and I immediately regretted being short with her. Maybe we should have done this differently. I could have taken the time to introduce myself and immodestly taken credit for saving the woman's life, have the relatives fawn around and worship me for the bizarre and heroic rescue. But this was Nick's case. He had already explained everything to the relatives. I didn't want to intrude, but I certainly didn't want to see the repair blown to pieces after all that effort. Having made the point, we wished them all a peaceful night and moved on. Sensitive souls, the intensive care doctors.

10 pm. Amir and I slipped silently into children's intensive care to check on the morning's case. Yet I was first drawn to the mother of the meningitis child whose black, gangrenous arms were now gone, replaced with rolls of pristine crepe bandage. Stark contrasts. Was she happy or sad that those mummified little hands had been removed? I wondered whether I would have asked to keep them had it been my child. I set that morbid thought aside and simply asked how the operation had gone. Was she, the mother, OK? Could I help her with anything? Fetch her a coffee? Anything at all to ease her pain? She just looked up at me with tears rolling down her cheeks

and said nothing. The nurse knew me well enough and shook her head. It was time to move on to my own little patient.

The chest drains were dry now, with a steady pulse and blood pressure. Nurse told me that Dr Archer had done an echo and was very pleased – no leak on either valve or across the patches. Fixed for life. The parents had drifted down from the ceiling after the shock of the sudden reoperation and had gone to crash out in their hospital room. They understood the difficulties we faced, which was what really mattered. Not the daily battle for the privilege of bringing a patient to the operating theatre, nor the repeated conflict over intensive care beds. As night fell, we hoped for stable patients, cheerful parents, happy husbands or wives, and a brighter future for them all. While they drifted off to bed, I strolled down a long, dark corridor to the doors of the accident department.

Out in the fresh air for the first time in sixteen hours, I stared at the night sky and waited for the ambulance to arrive. The operating theatre lay ready, the heart–lung machine was primed, and the team were watching *Newsnight* in the coffee room, yawning with boredom and resigned to the fact that we were likely to be there all night. My own thoughts drifted back to Gemma and the disappointment I must have caused her once again. But maybe I was wrong. Maybe she had a much better time without me.

11.50 pm. The ambulance with East Anglia Health Authority painted across the side finally arrived, its blue lights flashing. Paramedics threw open the rear doors and the long-off-duty Lucy stepped down the ramp. I just knew it was her. Like a scene from *Casablanca*, she walked towards the Emergency entrance carrying a stack of medical notes. I thought at that moment how beautiful she was.

'You're the Prof, aren't you?' she said. 'Mrs Norton told me about you. I trained in Cambridge and they still talk about you there.' Nothing positive, I expected.

The trolley bearing Steve's broken brain and body was being pushed towards us. The last time we met was barely six months before at a medical school reunion. He had delivered a very amusing speech celebrating the fact that all present were still alive despite his open heart surgery. I responded by jesting that things could have been different had he come to me for surgery. Now he was in Oxford in dire straits, not the next reunion we'd all anticipated, with his family still somewhere on the M25. I took his left hand, which firmly gripped mine. The good side that still moved. Then, along with Lucy, we walked in procession through the accident department down the corridor and straight into the operating theatres. A cursory glance at the CT scan confirmed the lethal diagnosis.

We can't operate without consent, but he was alone and I didn't want to be too explicit. I just told him that I would repair the dissection and with luck the stroke might recover. He struggled to tell me that he wanted to see Hilary and his children again before being put to sleep. Lucy had a number for Hilary, so I called. They were forty-five minutes away at best. Every extra minute meant less likelihood of neurological recovery, and too many hours had been wasted already. When I promised not to let him die, Steve used his left hand to mark a cross on the form. I counter-signed beneath, then Dave Pigott dispatched him to oblivion with a brain-protective barbiturate.

We had kept the interpersonal rapport to a minimum. Surgery has to be dispassionate, anonymous even. It was less of a problem because Steve couldn't speak and I simply couldn't verbalise the real risks to a friend who faced certain death if no one was prepared to operate. He was a doctor and knew the score. I didn't need to render him any more anxious in his last conscious moments.

I sat in the coffee room until the lily-white body had been painted brown with iodine and covered with drapes. I didn't want to see his flabby torso. I preferred to remember him the way he once was, that fine physical specimen striding out onto the pitch on a winter's afternoon, adrenaline pumping, ready for the scrap. Closely aligned in those days, we were very different characters now. Steve would sit in an office chatting affably to patients and dishing out pills. A proper doctor. There I was at midnight, ready to wield the knife and drive an oscillating saw through his chest, all after an endless day of disappointment, conflict and misery. But adrenaline dissipates the tiredness, wipes out time as the contest begins.

After the previous surgery, Steve had no pericardium or thymus gland between the back of the breast-bone and the front of his heart. So with an expanded, tissue-paper-thin aorta immediately beneath, chest re-entry with an oscillating saw was extremely hazardous. I reduced the risk of catastrophic bleeding by exposing the main artery and vein of the leg, and connecting them to the heart–lung machine. Should the saw lacerate the heart or aorta, I could go rapidly onto cardiopulmonary bypass, take pressure out of the circulation, then suck away blood from the bleeding site. Mostly that works. Sometimes it doesn't. If heart surgery were easy, everybody would be doing it.

Fixing Steve was like replumbing a Victorian house. All the main pipes were buggered and those coming out of the boiler needed to be replaced as they were rusty and might fall to bits at any moment, so I couldn't do it with hot water flowing through them. I needed the same conditions as fishbone lady – a cold brain and all the blood drained off into the machine. Dave put electroencephalogram leads onto the scalp to monitor the brain waves, which gradually disappeared as Steve's temperature fell but were already grossly abnormal after his stroke. Amir began by cutting the skin straight down the line of the scar from the previous operation, then used the electrocautery to sizzle through fat onto bone. He snipped through the old stainless-steel bone sutures with a wire cutter, then ripped them out. I was always going to open the sternum myself. Getting the depth of the oscillating saw just right is a matter of fine judgement. You must gently feel it pass through the back of the sternum, then pull back in case the posterior table of the bone and the muscle of the right ventricle are adherent.

The dissected aorta had the intimidating appearance of a tense aubergine, purple and angry, and I could see blood swirling beneath its perilously thin outer layer. Dave had positioned an echo probe in the oesophagus, directly behind the heart. This showed the original tear in the wall around 1 cm beyond the origin of the coronary arteries, the vital branches that supply the heart muscle itself. My job was to replace the torn part and redirect blood flow back to where nature intended, in the hope that this would restore flow to Steve's blocked brain and kidney arteries. The compromised kidney would undoubtedly survive, but the injured brain was unlikely to. It had been starved of blood and oxygen for too long, although barbiturates and cooling might help.

I told Brian the perfusionist to go onto bypass and cool to 18°C. Draining the whole living body of blood is a curious thing to do. Only vampires and the few heart surgeons who operate on congenital heart defects and extensive aortic aneurysms ever do it. I specialised in both, so I emptied people out on a regular basis. I once gave a spoof lecture about halal humans at Dracula's castle in Romania. I felt at home there. The Count and I had much in common.

I was normally relaxed about working against the clock, even when the brain had no blood flow. I didn't stand there contemplating the nerve cells as they died, nor did I rush the job. At 1.30 in the morning I told Brian to come off bypass and drain, the second time I had done that in twenty-four hours. Steve's cold, anticoagulated blood emptied into a reservoir and would sit there like a jug of Ribena until we pumped it all back again. I chopped away at the empty disintegrating aorta until I could see the inside of those vital branches coursing up into the head and arms.

The first step was to reapproximate the dissected layers of the filleted vessel with tissue glue. I was one of the first surgeons in the world to use the glue and it undoubtedly contributed to my gratifying survival rate. Then, with care bordering on obsession, I sewed in the vascular tube graft buttressed with strips of Teflon felt to prevent the stitches from cutting through the fragile tissue. Every patient's survival relied upon the connections between my cerebral cortex and fingertips, but this was especially the case in aortic dissections. Amir's eyes fixed on my every movement. He wanted to learn all the nuances of technique, which is why he willingly came in. Amir would definitely make it one day.

The repair to the aorta and inserting the graft without blood flow took thirty-four minutes. This lay within the window of safety for a normal brain, but Steve's brain was not normal. We carefully refilled the vascular tree with blood and evacuated air from the head vessels. Once back on cardiopulmonary bypass, blood oozed through the needle holes. These would continue to bleed until we reversed the anticoagulation that prevented blood from clotting on the foreign surfaces of the circuit. So many detailed steps to recall, but the whole sequence was ingrained in my neural circuits, with everything done on autopilot, even in the early hours of the morning.

It was now time to re-warm to normal body temperature. With warm blood coursing through his coronary arteries, Steve's heart muscle came to life again, first wriggling in what we call ventricular fibrillation, followed by spontaneous defibrillation and then the slow, lazy contractions that sped up as his temperature rose. Soon brain waves reappeared on the electroencephalogram. Dave thought it looked a bit better already.

The only other time that we watched this process of reanimation was when we tried to save children who had fallen through ice and drowned in a frozen pond, and there are rare cases of survival from Canada. Our Oxford trauma doctors pressed us to rewarm these lifeless bodies, and while we succeeded in salvaging hearts, lungs, livers and kidneys, the children were always fatally brain injured. We gave hope to their parents, then snatched it away again.

At 3 am I left Amir in charge at the operating table. Rewarming takes thirty minutes, and I'd been told that Hilary and several visitors were waiting in the intensive care relatives' room. On the positive side, their arrival broke the ice with our nursing staff and I at least now knew that there was a bed waiting for him. As I appeared in the doorway they all sprang to their feet. This was reflex not reverence. Here was a medical school reunion, such was Steve's popularity. Stan was a professor of oncology, John a consultant anaesthetist and Mike a GP. All were here to support Hilary and her children.

Before any type of greeting I told them the news they wanted to hear, that Steve's OK, I've repaired the aorta and fixed the blood supply to his brain. The surgery has gone well. This simple sentence scraped them down from the ceiling and untied the knot in their stomachs. News

– either good or bad – always dissolves that agonising fear of the unknown. As they stood there, far from home in the middle of the night, their old pal assumed a different persona. I was no longer the boozy buffoon from Scunthorpe.

There followed hugs, kisses and expressions of relief, then the usual request – 'Can we see him now?' I had to explain that Steve was still on the table with his chest wide open being rewarmed on the bypass machine and that while he was not entirely out of the woods, things had gone according to plan. I added that it was likely to be another couple of hours before we controlled the bleeding and closed him up. With that I left, intending to apologise to the sister in charge for springing this upon them. But it transpired that in fact there had been enough nurses – the last heart attack patient brought up from the catheter laboratory had ruptured his left ventricle and could not be resuscitated. The conveyor belt rumbled on.

I wandered wearily back to theatre and sat down with the two anaesthetists beside Steve's head. Amir was happy enough to remain in charge. Steve's temperature was back at 37°C and although still empty, his heart looked cheerful enough. I asked Brian to leave some blood in it, so any residual air would be ejected into the graft. I could hear Steve's artificial aortic valve clicking away reassuringly, and from the echo probe behind the heart we could see tiny bubbles flashing through it like a snow storm. I didn't have to ask. Amir already had the air needle in place. Bubbles fizzed out intermittently, then stopped. Now we were ready to come off the machine. I asked Dave to start ventilating the lungs and soon afterwards heard Brian say that he was 'off bypass'. Amir and the locum registrar stood like spectators at a football match, as I dispatched instructions from the stool. I was scrutinising the inside of the heart and aorta on the monitor screen while they watched it from the outside.

'How does it look?' I asked Amir. 'Any bleeding?'

'Looks great. Just some oozing from around the graft. Nothing serious.'

'What are you going to do now then?'

No answer. He was tired.

'Give the protamine,' I told Dave. Protamine extracted from salmon sperm reverses the anticoagulant effect of heparin, which comes from digested cow's guts. So my noble profession relied on cows and fish, a sobering thought at this time in the morning.

Amir gently packed gauze swabs around the heart to encourage the oozing blood to clot on them. Next he set about putting in the chest drains and stainless-steel wires to close up. The clock on the wall read 4.30. Dave flicked through a motorcycle magazine and Brian asked whether he could remove his equipment, get it ready for the morning and go home. No stamina, some people. Ayrin and her runner nurse were wilting too. I suggested they took turns to take a break while we transfused blood and clotting factors. For the first time a sense of calm filled the room. Job done.

Behind the operating theatre block was a car park, and beyond this lay Old Headington graveyard, thinly shielded by an unkempt hedge of privet and conifers. I walked out into the night past the Mercedes that never got to Cambridge, with Gemma's birthday present still concealed in the well of the passenger seat. I drifted on through the ornate metal gate to the brow of a hill overlooking the Oxfordshire countryside. There I lay silently on the grass by the grave of a baby girl and stared up into the night sky. The tombstone read, 'Taken too soon'. She'd been taken by me twenty years earlier, something I hadn't forgotten. She would have been Gemma's age now, had God not given her that twisted, convoluted heart that I failed to fix. So I sat with her from time to time when I was feeling bad, just to remind myself that I wouldn't always succeed. Difficult day today. Or was it yesterday?

6 am. Daylight broke the horizon and the sparrows chirped. Headlights sprinted around the Oxford ring road below, the early-bird London commuters and shift workers at the Cowley car plant. Sue would already be on her way into the office, so I ambled back to Theatre 5, now empty except for Ayrin. She was scrubbing blood and urine from the floor, ready for the morning's operating list. Steve was already settled in intensive care, surrounded by his extended family, perfectly stable.

Cheerful Amir said, 'Great case. So pleased you called me.'

The locum registrar was nowhere to be seen. Gone to collect his pot of gold, I thought.

I looked bad and smelled bad, so I went to the changing rooms, took a shower and stepped into clean theatre blues. The ritual signified the end of yesterday and the beginning of today. First, I made tea for Sue in the office, taking a dose of Ritalin with mine. Oxford students used the stimulant to aid concentration and inflate their exam grades; I used it for a boost when I was buggered or with added melatonin for jet lag. All in the patients' best interest, of course.

At 7.30 I joined the intensive care ward round. I related Steve's case story and asked whether his pupils were still small and reacting to light. Had anyone looked? Not yet, but they would. Had he shown any signs of waking up yet? No, but I was happy about that because I wanted him kept sedated and didn't want the tube in his windpipe to make him cough. Coughing would shoot his intra-cranial pressure through the roof and his brain was already too swollen in there. By explaining that to the juniors in front of Hilary, I assumed that they would get the message. At least I hoped they would.

I celebrated Steve's recovery with a sausage and egg sandwich, and, with the Ritalin kicking in, I felt better too. I had a floppy mitral valve to fix, and happily for me there was no bed for a second case. But the tone of day soon changed. As I emerged from theatre in the late morning, Steve partially woke from the sedation and started to struggle in his bed. With his brain swelling, he was disorientated, confused and agitated, then he started coughing vigorously against the tracheal tube and strained against the ventilator. He was a big man and not easy to control.

A debate ensued about whether to let him wake up fully and remove the endotracheal tube or re-sedate and paralyse him. In the midst of this, his left pupil dilated widely. Understanding its dire significance, John, our anaesthetist friend who had stayed by Steve's bedside, hurried off to find me in my office. We returned to check the pupils again. Steve's nurse thought that his right pupil was larger too. My spirits plummeted. I had hoped that cooling and barbiturates would limit the swelling around the stroke.

Did Hilary know of this sinister development? She had been given a relatives' room and gone there to rest after the stressful night. Perhaps it was best to leave the family alone until we gained a clear picture of what had happened. That meant an urgent brain CT scan, which was not easy for a post-operative patient connected to all the paraphernalia. Drips, drains, pacing wires and monitors had to be wheeled through the hospital corridors to the radiology department, then his paralysed body moved from his bed into the scanner. But without the pictures, we couldn't know how to help. So I walked round there myself and grovelled to my friend the chief radiographer to fit him in as a dire emergency.

As the scans emerged it was obvious that the whole brain was swollen. The parts damaged during the original stroke had haemorrhaged, probably as a result of the obligatory anticoagulant given during surgery. The injured brain had expanded like a sponge soaking up water yet confined in a rigid box. The skull has one hole at its base, through which the spinal cord enters its bony canal. When pressure rises, the brain stem can be forced down into the spinal canal with fatal consequences. This is called coning, and a blown pupil heralds that catastrophe. So I needed a brain surgeon to look at the scans with me.

It was not an easy conversation. Richard Kerr was the chief. He had seen it all, done it all, and was destined to be President of the British Association of Neurosurgeons. I asked him to decompress Steve's brain by removing the top of his skull. A craniectomy is like taking off the top of a boiled egg, except the bone is kept in a fridge and put back again should the patient survive. Richard was a man of few words. Before he even spoke, I knew he believed it to be a lost cause. I pleaded the family's case for them. Richard said that even if he survived, he would never be a GP again, indeed he might not even wake again. The delay in re-perfusing the stroke with the surgery had already destroyed his chance of survival. But that was now history. We couldn't turn the clock back.

So I played my last card. Steve was an old friend, I said, and I had spent all night and lots of money trying to save him. Richard groaned and went back through the scans.

'OK, you win. He has nothing to lose, but it has to be quick. I'll put off my next case.'

Within thirty minutes Steve was on a neurosurgery operating table at the far end of the hospital. I pushed the bed there myself.

2 pm. Steve's scalp was peeled back and the bone saw removed the top of his cranium, revealing a tense, swollen brain without pulsation. We were watching a dying brain. Richard inserted an intracranial pressure monitor into the pulp and closed the scalp skin loosely over the top. Then we took him back to cardiac intensive care, whose expertise he needed most.

Hilary and her children were still napping on a single bed and an armchair in their room. Consumed by my own misery and her husband's impending doom, I tentatively knocked on the door. Hilary read my gaunt expression and realised that this was not a social call.

'He's dead, isn't he?'

I hesitated to say no, since Steve's chances of survival were negligible. I just told her the truth. That he had a dilated pupil and the brain scan looked bad, that I'd immediately persuaded the finest neurosurgeon in the country to help, but we were both doubtful that Steve could recover now. It was a waiting game. More of our medical school friends arrived, hoping for better news. I heard that old chestnut – 'If anyone can save him, Westaby can.' But he couldn't. Great dissection repair, pity about the outcome. Soon afterwards, the second pupil dilated. Neither reacted to light. Despite the decompression, his brain was not going to recover. Hilary and the children had lost him.

Unbeknown to me, both Hilary and her eldest son had congenital polycystic kidneys, and the lad was teetering on the edge of needing renal dialysis. With remarkable composure, she asked whether he could be given his father's functioning kidney. An organ from his dad would provide the best possible chance of immune compatibility – same blood group, same genes, no rejection. For a brief moment I thought I could generate something positive out of this disaster. At the same time as the intensive care doctors carried out tests for brain stem death, I called the director of the transplant service.

What I learned was barely believable. While Steve was conscious he could have voluntarily donated a kidney to his son. Now that he was functionally dead, the family could request that he become an organ donor. But now the body blow. Whatever was still transplantable must go to the national donor pool. Those were the rules. The transplant authorities would not allow Steve's kidney to be used for his son, nor given to Hilary, who was close to needing a transplant herself. That was the law, so the Oxford transplant team couldn't get involved. I was dumbstruck, then apoplectic about it. Fucking bureaucracy.

Steve's ventilator was switched off at lunchtime. He died peacefully, surrounded by his family, with many of my medical school year grieving in the hospital corridors. I was alone in my office when his proud heart fibrillated, when the metallic click of his prosthetic valve finally came to a stop. Twelve hours earlier I had watched it beating vigorously and I had been confident that I'd saved him. Now it was forever still. All his organs died with him, except the corneas from his eyes. Despite my protestations, the transplant authorities had their way.

When Sue went home she left a note on my desk – 'The medical director wants to see you.'

'One day,' I said to myself, and drove home with Gemma's present still tucked away in the passenger seat.

Next day I was back in the car park by 6.10 am, another three cases on the operating list, beginning with a newborn infant whose right ventricle was missing. The car park lies between the graveyard and the mortuary at the back of the hospital. I always attended the autopsies of my own patients, so the morticians knew me well enough. This morning was a social call. I wanted to let Steve know that we had done our best for him. He was cold, pale and peaceful now. It was the only time I'd known him to be speechless. Had he still been able to talk, he would have said, 'You bastard. You were meant to get me out of this mess!' My instinct was to remove the drips and drains left in his lifeless body, but I was not allowed to. Those who die soon after surgery are the coroner's property, and the pathologists must satisfy themselves as to the cause of death. Not difficult in this case, but it was an autopsy I wouldn't be returning to watch. So I said my goodbyes to a great character.

There were many sad moments in my professional career, but this one stayed with me. Steve had devoted his life to the NHS but was caught up in the pass the parcel lottery that was out-of-hours surgery for aortic dissection. Eventually a decree was issued by the Society for Cardiothoracic Surgery that each regional centre must take responsibility for patients in their area. Special aortic dissection rotas were established in London and specific experienced surgeons designated to operate on the cases. That brought the mortality rate down. After UK Transplant prevented us taking a kidney for Steve's son, the issue of organ donation was not discussed further. A healthy liver and two lungs could have gone in to the pool, had that single functioning kidney been used in Oxford.

*   *   *

Later that year Steve's son Tom received a kidney donated by his wife. Steve's daughter Kate was given one of her husband's kidneys in 2015. Hilary was fortunate enough to meet a new partner and received one of his kidneys in 2011. They are all well.

3
risk

AS A BOY, MY STOICAL and religious parents taught me that I should never take risks – never to gamble with money, never to be deceitful or steal, never to cheat in exams. Not even to climb over the stadium wall to watch Scunthorpe United, because that was a form of stealing too. Consequently, I began life as both boring and introspective.

Eventually I learned that the ability to take risks is an indispensable part of human psychology. Victory in war depends upon risk-takers and recklessness, hence the adage 'Who dares wins'. The economy depends upon financial risk-takers. Innovation, speculation, even the exploration of the planet and outer space – all depend on putting something you cherish on the line in the hope of greater rewards. Thus risk-taking is the world's principal driver for progress, but it requires a particular character type, one defined by courage and daring, not reticence and prudence – Winston Churchill rather than Clement Attlee, Boris Johnson not Jeremy Corbyn.

In 1925, when Henry Souttar first stuck a finger into the heart and tried to relieve mitral stenosis, it posed a risk to his reputation and livelihood. When Dwight Harken removed a piece of shrapnel from a soldier's heart in the Cotswolds, it was a risk that went against all he'd learned from the medical textbooks of the day. By exposing blood to the foreign surfaces of the heart–lung machine, John Gibbon took a huge risk, as did Walton Lillehei with his reckless but brilliant cross-circulation operations, the only medical interventions in history outside the maternity ward that posed the risk of 200 per cent mortality. All progress in medicine and surgery is predicated on risk, yet I was taught to avoid it. Fortunately, things changed.

Character is said to be the product of nature and nurture, the former being the hand genetics deals to us. Then from birth onwards we are moulded by life's events. I started out well enough. My mother was an intelligent woman who was deprived of an education but read *The Times*. During the Second World War with the men away, she managed the Trustee Savings Bank on the High Street. One of my earliest recollections was that every birthday she took me, along with a bunch of flowers, to another woman's home. I thought that strange, but eventually I came to learn the significance of her pilgrimage.

After a long and painful labour my mother brought me safely back from the carnage of the delivery suite. She was exhausted, torn and bleeding, but elated to have a pink, robust son wailing from the depths of his newly expanded lungs. In the next bed, a wide-eyed factory girl was suffering noisily. Spurred on by the bossy midwife, she was preoccupied with pushing and pain. Finally, her perineum split. The straining emptied her uterus, bowels and bladder all at the same time, and the midwife caught the greasy, bloodied newborn like a cricket ball in the slips. The bonny little girl lay on a starched white towel soaked in urine, while the slithering umbilical cord was clamped and cut. Her baby's only dependable source of oxygen was now gone. Finally, the whole placenta separated and squelched out, to join the party in the outside world. Mother would need a gynaecologist to put things back where they should be – but not yet.

All babies are blue at birth, then they bawl as loudly as I did. It's cold outside and they no longer hear that soothing maternal heartbeat. Freed from their claustrophobic cocoon, they thrash their little arms and legs around and suck in air for the first time. At that point they should turn pink. This little mite stayed blue and silent. Listless, with eyes wide open but seeing nothing.

The midwife recognised that things were not right. She vigorously rubbed the baby's greasy back and swept her finger around its throat. Rough stimulation suddenly caused its breathing efforts to begin, but with a whimper not a roar. And the baby remained blue, a darker blue despite the rapid breathing, and still cool and limp. Now beginning to panic, the midwife called for an oxygen cylinder and some help. At first, the tiny oxygen mask helped. Baby's muscle tone improved but her grim slate blue colour persisted. The doctor arrived and listened to the tiny heaving chest with his stethoscope. There was a heart murmur, not loud but clearly audible when searching for something specific. It transpired that the artery to the lungs hadn't developed properly – pulmonary atresia, we call it. Dark blue blood returning from the tiny body streamed through a hole in the ventricular septum and back around the body. The chaotic circulation was progressively depleted of oxygen, accumulating more and more acid. The baby was doomed. A 'blue baby'. The doctor shook his head and walked away. Nothing could be done to help.

All this passed the mother by as she sweated in pain and perineal Armageddon. She was impatient to hold her new daughter. As they handed over the dying infant, the midwife's grave expression told the story, as did the child's pathetic face, lifeless and grey, eyes rolling aimlessly. Our factory girl pleaded for an explanation. Why so still and silent? Why not pink and warm like me in the cot next door? Milk started to flow, but there was no suckling. In 1948 blue babies died.

They returned to the maternity bed next to my mother. There was a stark contrast in mood after nine months of excitement and anticipation – one woman radiant, proud and optimistic with her robust, pink son, the other desolate with a grey, motionless little girl left to die in her arms. The curtains were pulled around. Her expectant husband was stuck at work, rolling steel, never to see his daughter alive. The hospital chaplain arrived as a matter of urgency to christen the child as life ebbed away. It was probably too late, but they went through the motions.

This emotional meltdown already greatly saddened my mother, then the contrasts deepened at visiting time when the families arrived. There were repeated emotional breakdowns as the young woman's parents, then the bereaved husband, arrived too late to see the dead baby before it was spirited away in a shoe box. Feelings of guilt quickly followed. What did she do wrong? Was it the cigarettes? Or was it the sickness pills? Should she have gone to church? My own family's joy was tinged with compassion for the poor girl. My mother stayed in the maternity bed beside her for five days while she was taken for pelvic surgery, with nothing to bring home but sadness and stitches.

The day was particularly sad because mother had read in her newspaper about a new blue baby operation in America, a miraculous procedure that could turn blue babies pink. Why had no one mentioned that? Surely the shiny new NHS, already three weeks old, could have managed to do the same. These grim memories never did fade. So it was that every birthday she took flowers in memory of the blue baby in the cot next to mine, a thoroughly decent thing to do on what should have been a happy day.

The story my mother recalled in *The Times* went something like this. At the Johns Hopkins Hospital in 1944, the children's heart doctor Helen Taussig challenged the chief of surgery Alfred Blalock to come up with a surgical solution for these doomed infants. Blalock's concept was that the subclavian artery that supplied blood to the baby's arm could be diverted into the chest and joined to the obstructed artery to the lungs. He anticipated that smaller collateral vessels around the shoulder blade would grow and keep the baby's arm supplied, as they did in animal experiments. The professor first attempted what became known as the Blalock–Taussig shunt in November that year. He was not a technically adept surgeon and had difficulty in joining the tiny blood vessels, yet to everyone's relief the operation immediately changed the child's colour from blue to pink, with an immediate resolution of breathlessness. What's more, the deprived arm continued to grow normally.

News spread fast about this transformational procedure. The pioneering British chest surgeon Sir Russell Brock – whose operating boots I inherited at the Brompton Hospital – invited Blalock and Taussig to demonstrate their operation in London. With no shortage of sickly blue babies, Blalock performed the shunt in ten consecutive infants without a single death, all the babies miraculously turning pink and beginning to grow. To conclude the visit, Blalock was invited to present his triumph in the Great Hall of the British Medical Association.

His lecture concluded with the room still darkened and silent following the projection of lantern slides. Suddenly a wartime searchlight traversed the length of the hall, its beam falling upon a Guy's nursing sister wearing her dark blue uniform with white linen cap and holding a blonde two-year-old girl. Days before, the little girl had been dying from cyanotic congenital heart disease. She was now pink following the new shunt procedure, and this theatrical effect prompted tumultuous applause from the audience. My mother's account of this story from *The Times* always resonated with me – quite simply, one of my earliest childhood recollections was of blue babies.

In the pioneering days after the blue baby operations, those who persisted then ultimately succeeded in operating on the heart undoubtedly had psychopathic tendencies. Could cardiac surgery in Europe really be possible? Probably, but there was still a long road ahead, one along which I was incongruously destined to travel from a very early age and was uniquely equipped to follow.

Most people have a dominant left cerebral hemisphere, which results in right-handedness and governs their language skills. In turn, the right cerebral hemisphere regulates spatial awareness, creativity and emotional responses. But I inherited a curious brain. I side-stepped lateralisation – an evolving process whereby different areas of grey matter adopt control of the various aspects of behaviour and skills – and developed co-dominant cerebral hemispheres, rendering me ambidextrous. Although I was predominantly right-handed through indoctrination at school, I could manipulate a pen, paint brush and eventually surgical instruments with both hands, and throw knots equally well with my left or right hand. I kicked a rugby ball with my left foot and batted left-handed at cricket.

Despite being totally useless at foreign languages, I possessed the innate ability to visualise the world in three dimensions. Manual dexterity paired with very precise spatial awareness made me a competent child artist and ultimately a natural surgeon. I painted landscapes of the steelworks of my native Scunthorpe lighting up the night sky, vivid red sunsets as the blast furnaces opened, courting couples kissing under the gas lamps and the steelworkers' grimy faces after a long day in the rolling mills. Unusual for a teenage boy, but crossed wiring makes people different.

Later in life, these innate skills enabled me to dissect the human body, then place every stitch in the right place first time, no faffing about. Precision of movement translates into economy of time. I became an effortlessly fast operator, although my hands never moved quickly. Of course, I had no understanding of this gift until I became a surgeon. Eventually I discovered that speedy operations were critically important in cardiac surgery – the shorter the procedure, the faster the patient's recovery.

At school I was known as the introverted artistic lad who wanted to be a doctor. But I wasn't particularly bright and would never secure a place at medical school these days. Bright pupils mastered maths and physics – I struggled, although I was good at biology and got by in chemistry. Ultimately it was my sheer determination to escape the dilapidated streets and terraced council houses that found me reading medicine in London, the fish out of water who wanted to be a heart surgeon when he grew up.

It was my attempt to fit in with the public school crowd that compelled me to play rugby and drink beer. I had all the requisite skills to kick and throw the stupidly shaped ball. In fact, I was rather good at it, rapidly ascending from a clueless beginner in the 4th XV to a regular spot in the 1st. For a so-called caring profession, London hospitals rugby was outrageously physical and violent. At its peak in the late 1960s, a Guy's player captained

England and the legendary fullback J. P. R. Williams played for St Mary's and won his first Welsh cap in 1969. General George S. Patton once remarked, 'I don't measure a man's success by how high he climbs but how high he bounces when he hits bottom.' As a wing forward I tried to tackle Williams during a Hospitals' Cup game at Richmond and took a battering for my efforts. Yet with bruised ribs and a bloody nose I finally succeeded.

My most serious injury was yet to come. It happened on a rugby club tour to Cornwall at the end of my second term. I have absolutely no recollection of the incident myself, so the explanations came later. We were confronted by a team of hefty Cornish farmers on a muddy, wind-swept pitch in Penryn. I had just prevented an opposition try with an outrageously high tackle that inevitably provoked retaliation. The loose scrum broke up and the players ran to scramble after the ball. I was left prostrate and senseless face down in a puddle following a targeted boot to the head. It was some time before these caring medical students came back for me, and by then I was blue.

When I came round again I was staring at a dim light-bulb that seemed brighter than the sun. All around were my equally dim medical school teammates, ready to cart me off to the bar instead of a hospital. As in boxing, a knockout wasn't uncommon in student rugby, and we still had some serious drinking and singing to do. The touring tradition was that we entertained the local yokels with merriment and senseless dirty lyrics as only the London medical students could. Our lodgings were miles away in

St Ives, so despite the headache from hell and a light show that resembled New Year's Eve over the Thames, I had little alternative but to join in.

Next morning I was difficult to rouse. Steve Norton, a well-meaning friend, gave me a gentle shake, and I responded by projectile vomiting over his legs. My head hurt and the winter sunlight burned my eyes – photophobia of the worst kind – so I dived back under the blanket. Half an hour later the local doctor arrived. He was a good old-fashioned GP who took my pulse and blood pressure, then attempted to inspect the back of my eyes with an ophthalmoscope. These three observations were sufficient. I was in deep trouble. Slow pulse rate, high blood pressure and swollen optic discs. In addition, there were tell-tale comma-shaped bruises beneath both eyes. Everything pointed to a battered, swollen brain that last night's beer didn't help. The doctor berated my clueless teammates, sent for an ambulance and dispatched me to the neurological unit at Truro Hospital. This spelled the end of my jolly tour and, as I subsequently learned in London, it could have heralded the end of my medical career. Bizarrely, it had quite the opposite effect.

The skull X-rays revealed a hairline crack in the frontal bone, so, as thick as my skull appeared to be, the kicking had fractured it. The obvious signs of raised intracranial pressure went along with that. A gruff brain surgeon from Plymouth was in the hospital for an outpatient clinic and came to check me out. Treatment meant an intravenous drip with mannitol solution to draw water from my swollen brain, along with a urinary catheter and bag to cope with the diuresis. He wanted to take me back to Derriford Hospital for an intracranial pressure monitor, but I abjectly refused to go. The pipe in my penis was bad enough. I didn't want a hole drilled in my skull and a bolt in my brain too. This stroppy lack of cooperation was a sign of things to come. I was agitated and overtly aggressive, no longer the mild-mannered, sensitive lad who had travelled down to Cornwall. There were no CT scans back in 1967, so there could be no direct images of my traumatised cerebral cortex. But something had definitely changed. Everyone expected me to revert to normal when the swelling abated. Fortunately for me, I didn't.

Truro shipped me back to Charing Cross Hospital, where they admitted me to a quiet single room on a surgical ward overlooking the Strand. That same night I tried to seduce a pretty staff nurse, who responded by giving a sharp tug on my urinary catheter. The rapid displacement of the restraining balloon from bladder to prostate gland was enough to quell my ardour for one night, although the memory didn't last. I was soon at it again.

The following day I was surrounded by student nurses who knew me from the Friday-night dances. Then my teammates brought in *Playboy* magazines and bottles of beer that they hid in the commode. It felt as if I were being treated like royalty. A bespectacled Harley Street neurologist in customary morning suit came to assess the injured medical student. I remember thinking that he looked like a penguin. When asked what I remembered about the whole episode I impolitely answered, 'Bugger all, I'm afraid!', backstreet language that I would never normally use in the company of a senior consultant. This clearly amused him and helped confirm his impressions about the severity of the injury. He tested every reflex and movement and, while noting my crossed wiring, declared my motor skills to be intact. He then sent along a psychologist. She did more tests, then decided to give me a tutorial about the consequences of frontal brain injury.

She explained that the right cerebral hemisphere is the home of critical reasoning and those thought processes involved in the avoidance of risk-taking. The crack in my skull was directly over the right frontal cortex, so the brain swelling probably explained the lack of inhibition, irritability and occasional aggression reported by the staff looking after me. I thought I had been polite and nice to the Charing Cross nurses, but maybe not. Some of her tests suggested that I scored highly on something called the 'psychopathic personality inventory'.

'But don't worry,' she said, 'most high achievers are psychopaths, particularly surgeons.' She then went on to explain my temporary change in personality using a classical case study that they use to teach psychology students.

In 1848 Phineas Gage was the foreman of a crew of construction workers in the American Midwest who were excavating rocks to make way for a railroad track. This involved drilling holes deep into boulders, then filling them with dynamite. A fuse was inserted and the hole plugged with compacted sand using a tamping iron. During the process a spark between metal and rock ignited the explosive, causing the four-foot iron rod to be propelled at high speed through Gage's skull. Having entered beneath the left cheek bone, it exited the scalp and was recovered thirty yards from the accident. Gage didn't even lose consciousness. He simply climbed into an ox cart and headed off to seek medical assistance. The local physician, Dr Harlow, removed shards of bone and replaced larger skull fragments, then covered the wounds with adhesive tape.

Gage's brain unfortunately became infected with fungus and he lapsed into a coma. The family prepared a coffin for him, but Harlow operated, releasing eight fluid ounces of pus from under the scalp wound. Miraculously he recovered and within weeks had regained 'full possession of his reason'. But his wife and those close to him recognised sinister changes in his disposition, which Harlow described in the *Bulletin of the Massachusetts Medical Society*.

> He is fitful, irreverent, indulging at times in the grossest profanity which was not previously his custom, manifesting but little deference for his fellows, impatient of advice when it conflicts with his desires, at times pertinaciously obstinate yet capricious and vacillating ...

In this regard, his mind was changed so decidedly that his acquaintances said he was 'no longer Gage'.

Clearly that story resonated with me. I had sustained damage to the prefrontal cortex, which could cause personality changes while leaving other higher neurological functions intact. Yet I denied the fact that I was in any way different. Poor Gage lost his job and ended up displaying himself along with the tamping iron in Barnum's Circus in New York. After dying during a seizure at the age of thirty-five, he was buried in San Francisco. Soon after, his unscrupulous brother-in-law exhumed the body, and Gage's skull and the tamping iron are still on display at Harvard Medical School.

At that point I felt that the nice psychologist was gently trying to tell me something like 'Go back to Scunthorpe and join the circus.' When my brain swelling abated, I did head home for the Easter holidays, leaving my poor parents baffled as to the unexpected effects of a medical school education. Then I returned more determined than ever to resume my medical studies.

While I wouldn't recommend head trauma as a career-enhancing strategy, what that head injury did for me in the medium term was quite extraordinary. In place of the wilting violet, I became disinhibited, bold and egotistical – no more exam anxiety nor embarrassment when called upon to speak in front of a crowded lecture theatre. Within weeks I had become the wildly extrovert compere for the students' Christmas show, social secretary for the medical school, then cricket captain … and so it went on. I seemed immune to stress and now became a habitual risk-taker, an adrenaline junkie who constantly craved excitement. Personal problems that I used to dwell upon for days were swept aside. In short, I emerged from the head-injury experience both disinhibited and ruthlessly competitive. Born with both the coordination and manual dexterity to become a surgeon, I had now acquired the necessary personality traits as well. Yet I never lost my empathy, that element of emotional intelligence enabling us to appreciate the feelings of others, the ability to care about people that all doctors and nurses are meant to have, although many don't.

With the introduction of magnetic resonance imaging it became possible to visualise brain networks within the cerebral cortex. The frontal lobes sense then process danger or fear by relaying scary stuff to the amygdala deep within the brain. Psychopaths lose the connection between the two, and characteristically manifest ruthless-ness and disregard for authority. Two psychologists named Blumer and Benson wrote about the personality changes of traumatic prefrontal cortex injury, describing the syndrome as 'pseudo-psychopathy'. Head-injury patients may show lack of inhibition or restraint, failure to appreciate risk, impatience and diminished guilt, but without the loss of compassion that characterises the inherent psychopath. That was me in a nutshell, although I had no insight into it at the time.

I was in New York City when I first registered the reck-less absence of fear that enabled me to live life out on the edge. There is a saying – 'Courage is not the absence of fear but the willingness to face it.' It was 1972, and as part of a medical students' scholarship at the Albert Einstein School for Medicine I was working a night shift in the emergency room of Morrisania Hospital in Harlem. In the gloom of the early hours the whole department was struggling with the consequences of drug abuse and gang warfare. A young nurse tried to confiscate some contaminated syringes from a drug-crazed addict who had been wounded in a fight. He went berserk with a flick knife and tried to kill her. I saw this coming and went for him before he reached her, a full-on rugby tackle sending the two of us sailing over the chairs in the waiting room.

The addict's knife sliced open the thumb of my right hand and blood splattered in streaks over my pristine white intern's vest, but the set-to didn't last for long. One of the guards hit my combatant over the head with a riot stick and he ended up in neurosurgery. The grateful chief nurse stitched my wounds, then I went to watch the burr holes being drilled in the lad's skull. And believe it or not I felt sorry for him. I felt sad for his miserable life.

A report was sent back to the medical school about my heroism. But in reality it was actually less than heroic, because I simply didn't need courage to face it. It did, however, bring me the glittering prizes. 'The student most likely to succeed', then the prestigious residency posts for both the professor of medicine then the professor of surgery. Did the head injury stop me playing rugby? Not at all. I just became even more aggressive.

Psychopathy is widely acknowledged in the surgical world. As recently as 2015 the *Bulletin of the Royal College of Surgeons* published an article entitled 'Are surgeons psychopaths? And if so, is that such a bad thing?' The authors argued that complete emotional detachment from the fraught discussions surrounding life-or-death decisions resulted in better choices being made. While this sounds reasonable, the dictionary describes psychopaths as cold-hearted, grandiose and overconfident, with an overblown sense of self-worth and capable of 'blame externalisation' by dismissing culpability and failing to exhibit remorse. Certainly, that description fits well with other accounts of the surgical stereotype, and of risk-takers in the financial world.

But when the risk-taker in medicine wins, everyone else does too. We have to be kept free to experiment and push the boundaries, just as our predecessors did. But I fear that this has now all gone. Risk management is a substantial industry these days and the regulatory authorities are such that everyone strives for a risk-free environment. Even our so-called clients are routinely risk stratified, with the implication that while it is not satisfactory to terminate a low-risk candidate, bumping off the odd high-risk patient is excusable. What a miserable way to view any profession.

I never looked upon surgery that way. I attracted high-risk cases like a magnet, then revelled in the contest, me versus Grim Reaper. I was repeatedly told that my schemes would never work – that silicone rubber tubes in the windpipe would clog (they didn't); that pulseless people couldn't survive (they did); that putting electricity into people's heads was dangerous (it wasn't); that injecting stem cells directly into scarred hearts would cause sudden death (not so; we use them to treat heart failure now). Risk-taking is a vital part of medical innovation, and life itself is a risk. If deprived of the opportunity to innovate, cardiac surgery is finished.

4

hubris

THROUGH THAT RETROSPECTOSCOPE I viewed the next stages of my career with deep embarrassment. I wasn't born an egotistical maniac. In my youth I had been a shy, caring grammar-school boy who wanted to help people. Until that peculiar quirk of fate on a Cornish rugby pitch I lacked confidence. Afterwards, the pendulum swung way over in the opposite direction. My self-belief and unbridled enthusiasm were rarely tempered by the fact that there was a human life at the sharp end of my scalpel. That didn't register. In short, I was out of control.

My post-traumatic boldness and lack of inhibition repeatedly got me into trouble. Had my personality not been so far towards the timid end of the spectrum beforehand, I might have ended up like Phineas Gage, unemployable and potentially criminal. As it was, I was simply regarded as an unflappable, overconfident and ruthlessly ambitious young man who could operate. I was bored easily, neglected paperwork, drove too fast and left my little blue sports car anywhere that suited me.

I was also an opportunist. While working as a junior doctor in the Liver Unit at King's College Hospital in London, I learned that the senior registrars were travelling to Cambridge to supervise the post-operative care for Professor Roy Calne's pioneering liver transplants. These were young physicians well into their training who had absolutely no interest in surgery, let alone staying up at night to watch blood drip relentlessly into drainage bottles. One weekend when no one else was prepared to do it, I volunteered and ventured up to Addenbrooke's Hospital. This was my opportunity to watch a liver transplant over the great man's shoulder, albeit under the pretence of gaining a better understanding of what was required afterwards. The strategy paid off. The patient recovered without any complications and everyone thought that I was another Liver Unit senior registrar.

The Cambridge surgical training rotation was the most prestigious in the country and I loved the city. Only childhood introspection and an ingrained inferiority complex had stopped me from accepting an offer to study medicine at the university. My Jekyll and Hyde transformation changed all that. When the next surgical posts were advertised, I applied and gave my references from Charing Cross and the Brompton. On the basis of my work with his transplant patients, Professor Calne waved me through. Apart from my Brompton adventures and a few appendicectomies done as a house officer in London, I had no practical surgical experience, but that made little difference in those days. What mattered was the confidence – indeed, the recklessness – to just get on and operate. I threw myself into the job and like a dog cut my teeth on bones. It's hard to kill people during orthopaedic surgery, although not quite impossible.

Over an icy Christmas period in 1976 I lived in the hospital and operated on more than a hundred fractured hips in the elderly after falls. Two of them died just because the stress of surgery was too much for them. The over-nineties are difficult to mobilise after surgery, so they lie in bed, get pneumonia, then Grim Reaper calls. But we can't just put them down or leave them in pain, so we go through the motions. After six months of human carpentry and gruesome trauma calls I had mastered the basics – simple stuff like handling the instruments, stopping bleeding and having the balls to operate independently without having to call for help – and I revelled in the great romance of learning to be a surgeon. Next came general surgery, full-blown blood-and-guts stuff, especially when on call at night. I soon acquired the nickname 'Jaws' because of the short time it took me to amputate a leg.

In the 1970s there was no medication to cut down stomach acid, so every night brought perforated duodenal ulcers with peritonitis, or exsanguinating stomach bleeding. Then there was intestinal obstruction through bowel cancer, or traumatic injuries to the liver or spleen. The more dramatic the problem, the better I liked it. I operated all day and most of the night, and my bosses were happy for me to do so. Except for one tedious issue that I blamed on attention deficit disorder – I never got around to the paperwork. Patients' notes piled high in the registrars' room, waiting for discharge summaries or letters to the GP. Benign retribution went unheeded, so I was eventually banned from the operating theatres until I had cleared the lot.

Late one Saturday evening, 'Jaws' was called to see an eight-year-old girl brought in by ambulance with sudden severe abdominal pain. Her parents were Jehovah's Witnesses who were clearly concerned about the prospect of her needing surgery. She had a bit of a temperature and generalised abdominal tenderness, worse over the site of her appendix. Common things are common. I informed the parents that she had signs of peritonitis and I thought her appendix might have ruptured. I needed to take her to theatre immediately, whip out the useless worm and give her belly a washout. They asked whether she would lose any blood.

'Absolutely not. It will be all done in fifteen minutes.'

Already they had the utmost confidence in me, given the straightforward and unequivocal advice.

'And we won't even think about testing her blood group,' I assured them.

I went off to theatre, with an anaesthetic registrar and the houseman on call to assist me. This was the last case in line for surgery, and there was a party waiting for us all in the nurses' quarters. I made a small gridiron incision in the right iliac fossa directly over the usual location of the appendix. When I reached the transparent peritoneal lining of the abdominal cavity, I expected to see straw-coloured fluid before lifting out the inflamed wiggly appendage with a hole in the end. Not this time. It was dark in there. When I tented up the membrane with forceps and nicked it with scissors, fresh blood spilled out.

I got that sinking feeling. I had thought she looked pale because she felt bad.

'Did we get the haemoglobin and white blood cell count back yet?' I asked my anaesthetist.

'Not yet. Why?'

'Because the fucking peritoneum is full of blood.'

The anaesthetist's head appeared swiftly over the top of the blood–brain barrier, that green drape hanging on drip poles that keeps their nose out of the wound because they never bother to wear masks.

'Shit, what's going on?' he said.

He told the anaesthetic nurse to fetch blood from the fridge and frantically started measuring the blood pressure: 100/70, pulse rate 105. I immediately made it clear that we would get sued if we gave blood without first raising the issue with the parents. They would certainly refuse it.

He wanted the on-call consultants. I didn't. I wanted to find out what was wrong and fix it myself. I remained irrationally calm and made a second, much larger incision in the midline of the belly. More blood spewed out. By then, my rational colleagues had become ditherers who needed to abrogate responsibility as quickly as possible. Quite reasonably, they thought she might be an abused child and that this was trauma to the liver or spleen. But if that were the case, there should be bruising on the skin, together with other evidence over the rest of her body.

What did I feel? Just curiosity and excitement, because this had to be something rare. My prefrontal cortex should have been dispatching messages of alarm and anxiety to the amygdala, but I'd left fear on the pitch in Penryn. I was there to score points and prove that I was the most competent of the registrars. What was that assessment from medical school? 'The one most likely to succeed. Brave but lacking insight.' Not my fault, as I would have to explain on numerous occasions until I became a consultant myself.

I dragged the intestines out through the incision to search for the major blood vessels. Logically, if any of these had been pissing blood the girl would never have reached hospital. Intuition told me that the initial bleeding had already stopped, as her blood pressure and pulse rate were now stable. I inspected the liver and spleen but they were blameless, so I ruled out injury. Next, I worked through the gut inch by inch, finally locating the problem not far from where the appendix should have been. It was a vanishingly rare congenital anomaly that I would never encounter again, a ruptured duplication cyst of the large bowel. I identified a few residual bleeders and dealt with them with the sizzling electrocautery. I could now tell the rest of the team that the bleeding was under control. The girl was safe ... so relax.

'What are you going to do about the duplication cyst?' asked the emotionally drained anaesthetic registrar, whose boss was on the way in.

'Cut out the bloody colon,' I snapped, somewhat irritated by his persistent feebleness. 'Why don't you go and be a GP?'

A nonsensical rhyme drifted back and forth through my disinhibited brain: 'Pass the gas, then kiss my ass!' I tied off the relevant blood vessels, clamped the slithering guts, then chop, chop, out it came. I joined the two ends with an obsessional continuous stitch, then washed blood and shit out of the peritoneal cavity with warm saline solution. Suck it all out and close up the two incisions. Job done. It was really just plumbing, when all the angst and empathy were set aside.

By then the consultant anaesthetist had arrived. With crass disregard for seniority I asked what had kept him, as I cheerfully sewed up the skin. The first thing anaesthetists do is to peer over the top of the drapes and ask whether everything is under control. So I reached over to the specimen bucket and proudly presented the offending pathology.

'Never heard of it,' he said.

'Neither have I. It must be rare. What's the blood pressure now?'

'100/70.'

'And pulse?'

'100.'

'Did you get a haemoglobin yet?'

'It's 10.'

'Good enough,' I concluded. 'She's safe now.'

The consultant politely enquired whether I had let my paediatric boss Mr Dunn know about the case.

'No time,' I lied. 'I thought the girl was still bleeding and Mr Dunn's at a college dinner. I'll surprise him on the ward round in the morning.'

I now needed to explain to the girl's parents why she had both an appendix incision and a bloody great scar down her middle, and why it hadn't been the fifteen minutes I had told them to expect. As with all parents waiting for news about their child's surgery, they were in meltdown by this stage. My broad grin in the doorway of the waiting room told them all they needed to know – their daughter was safe, despite my incorrect diagnosis.

I switched from psychopathic cerebral cortex to defensive and compassionate cerebral cortex, which earned me a generous present when the girl left hospital. Like my willingness to help Down's syndrome children, I always looked after Jehovah's Witness patients in the coming years. At least they have solid values and a religion that doesn't hurt anyone. They sometimes left theatre with a haemoglobin level one third of normal, but they usually recovered.

Professor Calne encouraged me to play rugby for the local team and get my name in the newspapers – the crazy wing forward who scored the tries. When I walked into the operating theatre or charged out onto a rugby pitch, the psychopathy switch was thrown on. And the injuries kept coming. During one game, a metal stud tore through my scalp, leaving a 12 cm groove in my skull. I insisted on going back to Cambridge where Sarah, the nurse who would eventually become my wife, was on duty in the accident department. I asked her to stitch me up and give me a tetanus jab, but not to bother with the local anaesthetic. Soon I was screaming pathetically for it.

Then came the fractured jaw at Christmas, when I ended up opening a motorcyclist's chest in the accident department. I was still wearing my rugby kit, covered in mud, spitting my own blood into the scrub sink, but I was right there in the waiting room and there was no other surgeon in the hospital who could try to save him. I then did a stupid thing by declining surgery for my own jaw fracture, after which I had to endure monster doses of intramuscular penicillin injected into my backside to prevent infection in the bone. The nurses revelled in using my arse as a pin cushion. Ultimately it was this injury that helped me pass the miserable Royal College of Surgeons final examination. I could barely speak in the oral tests, so there was none of the bravado and bullshit that had failed me the first time round.

I left Cambridge replete with qualifications and priceless surgical experience. I was as confident as I possibly could be, but carrying way too much emotional baggage. Lack of inhibition promotes sexual promiscuity and its fair share of trouble. The *Oxford English Dictionary* associates psychopathy with 'disinhibition and callous lack of concern for others'. It certainly goes with little blue sports cars and an inflated ego.

The Hammersmith Hospital and Royal Postgraduate Medical School invited me to take a post as cardiac surgical trainee during my last few weeks at Addenbrooke's. This obviously came as a pleasant surprise. Perhaps the job had been advertised and there were no suitable applicants, but I was still pleased to be asked. The euphoria didn't last long, however, as I was soon irritated by constantly having to assist putty-fingered senior registrars who struggled to stitch the beating heart. It is slippery, moves constantly, and I was convinced I could do better myself. As I became progressively more stroppy about assisting and not wielding the knife myself, I was dispatched to the chest surgery limb of the rotation at Harefield Hospital, which had all the appeal of a wet weekend in Scunthorpe, something I was far too familiar with. Lungs just inflated and deflated – not very challenging. So I went AWOL.

I saw a job advertised for a locum consultant general surgeon in Hong Kong. Intriguingly, it was with the island's oldest medical practice, involved operating in two private clinics on the Peak, and while the resident surgeon was away on sabbatical the successful applicant would have use of his apartment, his Porsche and membership of the Hong Kong Club. This was an opportunity to put my glittering Cambridge experience to the test on the other side of the world in a completely different culture. And why not? When I was given the job, I demanded three months' leave from the cardiac rotation and took off. It was a gamble, but I was frustrated and restless in London, verging on the self-destruct mode. Ultimately, it saved me from being thrown out.

At the Canossa and Matilda hospitals I worked single-handed, with Roman Catholic nuns as assistants. No registrars or housemen to help here. But the nuns brought a sense of calm and harmony to an operating theatre. After all, who could rant and rave at the Holy Sisters? Better still, they were experienced and trustworthy to an

extent rarely found at home. Their job was to assist the
surgeons, and they kept my roving eye focused on the task
at hand. Even I couldn't flirt with a nun. In turn, I was
eager to impress and to instil them with confidence in the
young upstart from England.

An opportunity to do just this arose sooner than I
might have wished. The practice gastroenterologist
referred a nineteen-year-old Chinese girl to me with a
problem I had never encountered in the West. The slightly
built but beautiful young woman from a wealthy Chinese
family had come along with bleeding from the back
passage. Surely it must be haemorrhoids, but the gut
doctor's well-educated index finger had located a mass in
the rectum. Rectal cancer at nineteen? I didn't believe the
referral letter, but apparently a biopsy had already
confirmed it. I met with the devastated girl and her mother
in my outpatients' clinic at the Peninsula Hotel, across on
the Kowloon side via the bustling Star Ferry.

In those days the only treatment for a low tumour in
that part of the bowel was to radically excise the rectum
and leave the patient with a lifelong colostomy stoma. For
a teenage Chinese girl, voluntary euthanasia would have
been preferable. I was cautioned by the nuns about that
when I discussed whether I could do what we call an
abdominoperineal resection. Two experienced surgeons
would usually operate together, one mobilising the rectum
from above through an incision in the abdomen, the other
working up to the tumour from below after excising the
poor girl's anus. I needed to think carefully. Should I take
this on myself or refer the girl on to an experienced team

at the University Hospital? As usual I felt that I was the man for the job, even though I had never done the procedure before. How stupid and deluded was that? Which mattered most – my reputation or the girl's life?

When I first met the family the mother wasn't prepared to let me examine her daughter and they clearly didn't want surgery. I immediately felt desperately sorry for the girl. Next to surgeons, children's cancer doctors score highest on the psychopathy scale and I can understand why. Human nature normally cannot tolerate witnessing such angst in young people or their parents on a daily basis. Through a Cantonese translator I confronted the mother with a harsh question. Was she prepared for her daughter to die a horrible death from cancer merely because the colostomy bag might destroy her marriage prospects? This abrupt provocation broke through the ethnic barrier and made her cry, so I apologised, something they didn't expect from a bullish Western surgeon.

I simply had to keep talking until I persuaded them that the English doctor could cure her cancer. In fact, the gods had persuaded me to fly from London to do just that. As they left I genuinely believed that I would never see them again. There was an element of relief in that. I feared that the girl would terminate her own life rather than bring shame on her family. Shame merely for being dealt that genetic self-destruct button. But they did come back, so I had to face up to it. Was I anxious? No. Was I concerned by the extent and complexity of abdominoperineal resection? Certainly. I had seen a few, although a long time ago. But I was sure it would all come back to me once I got started.

Barely a word was said during the five-hour operation. Occasionally I had to ask for an instrument. The correct implement was robotically slapped into my palm, as if by remote control. There was the occasional 'Oh shit' or 'Bugger', and a constant trickle of perspiration down my back. The nuns moved the lights and – straight out of good old medical movies – mopped my brow. Thankfully the liver was clean, with no sign of the tumour having spread. For once I moved slowly and deliberately through tiger country, mobilising the colon from above, then the rectum behind her uterus. As a budding heart surgeon, this was the first and last time I would do it, so I wanted it to be a success. Most of all I needed to get the site of the colostomy right. This is where the colon and its contents would forever emerge from the abdominal wall. It had to be neat like a rose bud and in the perfect spot so as not to interfere with her clothes.

Although the combination of incisions was excruciatingly painful for her, she recovered rapidly, as only the young can. I was able to reassure the family that there was no obvious sign of tumour spread. Then the pathologist's microscope indicated that there was no invasion of tumour right through the bowel wall or into the lymph nodes. Nor did she experience any complications. The nuns said that they were proud of me – I was exceptionally proud of myself, happier than I had been after any operation, and thoroughly relieved for myself and that family.

That night I had a few drinks at the enigmatic Hong Kong Club, then sat alone in the haze of the sauna. Time after time my brain worked backwards through the steps of the operation. Should I have risked it in the first place? What was more important to me? Demonstrating to myself that I was invincible, or that poor girl's safety? It was a career-defining moment. While I still had no fear, my insight was returning. Hong Kong put my own privileged existence in perspective. Working alongside the nuns and sharing some of my own problems with them restored an inner peace that I had lost several years before.

It was then that I started to operate on chests in the public hospital in Kowloon. Lung cancer was common there and there was no one else to do it. I treated traumatic injuries, drained pus and corrected chest deformities in children, all on a philanthropic basis, which restored my self-respect. Unexpectedly I found myself sticking my index finger into hearts to relieve rheumatic mitral stenosis because it was that – or nothing at all.

The more I took on, the more they wanted me to do, and I revelled in it. They wanted me to stay, and I was certainly tempted. Chinese patients didn't complain about their lives, nor did their surgeons. They did the best they could with what they had, and much of this was a throwback to the previous century. Instead, I resolved to begin all over again in England and use what I had learned on the other side of the world. I would try to be less arrogant and detached, perhaps less of a loner, although none of this would be easy.

*   *   *

I hadn't been long back at the Hammersmith before I was in trouble again, and I was already close to being ejected from the training rotation for disappearing for three months. Same shit, different day. This time I had taken a stab wound of the heart to the operating theatre without telling the consultant on call. 'So what?' I thought to myself. 'The man was dying. I saved him and prevented a murder.' I argued that there had been no time to get in touch with him on the way to theatre because my mind was on the business in hand. But that was not the point. However confident I was of my abilities, there was always protocol to be followed. So much for my Chinese New Year resolutions. I was a recidivist, undisciplined and evidently uncontrollable.

After the stab wound, Professor Bentall, whose eyes and hands were not what they used to be, adopted me as his personal assistant. I would do the surgery, he would assist, even for his overseas private patients. I could certainly operate, no one doubted that. My temperament was the issue – the rough edges, the blatant disregard for authority and lack of insight still lingered after my skull fracture. I had morphed into a ruthlessly ambitious prat who needed to be reined in or chucked out. One or the other. Remaining the same was not sustainable in an NHS hospital. Hong Kong was one thing, Du Cane Road W12 quite another.

One morning, after parking my blue MG in the hospital manager's space outside the main entrance, Professor Bentall called me to his office. I anticipated a complaint from on high and a bollocking for yet another misdemeanour. I would respond with Communist China stuff about equality and what really mattered in life. But no. There had been a complaint, of course, but it simply precipitated a conversation that had long been in the offing. He could see that I was still not happy. Did I want to go to America and work with some of the big names? I didn't need to think about that. I just said yes. I would go to California and work with Norman Shumway, the heart transplant pioneer.

That was not at all what Bentall had in mind. He was magnanimous enough to acknowledge my surgical potential but re-emphasised the fact that I was completely off the rails. If I went to Stanford, I would only get worse. I should go to John Kirklin, the well-known disciplinarian, who had moved from the Mayo Clinic to establish the world's foremost academic surgical programme at a new hospital in Birmingham, Alabama. The steamy Deep South. Prof had already spoken to him about me. Kirklin would sort me out, then I could return to a senior post at the Hammersmith. This was a take it or leave it ultimatum. So I took it. That was my only option. I was notorious in the specialty, mostly for the wrong reasons. But remember, it wasn't my fault. It was those buggered-up brain pathways. Hopefully they would regenerate one day, but hopefully not too soon. I had succeeded in China. Could I emulate that in Alabama?

5

perfectionism

29 DECEMBER 1980. THE GREAT WRENCH. Leaving behind the car crash of my personal life, and my precious young daughter, Gemma, I set out for Birmingham, Alabama. This was make-or-break time for my career prospects as a cardiac surgeon. My wild antics and derisory approach to the surgical training programme had ruffled too many feathers in London. Now I needed to make it in America. My scholarship in New York had given me some insight as to what to expect, but the Deep South was different, hot and steamy in ways other than the weather.

For me, 1981 had to be about change. It was high time for the caterpillar to morph into a butterfly, then protect his wings from being singed in the fire. Heart surgery was evolving continuously, with rapidly improving results. The cavalier approach of 'Let's give it a go and see if the patient makes it' had passed. It wasn't manual dexterity or operative technique that now made the difference, it was surgical science. To operate inside the heart, the organ has to be flaccid and still. This can only be achieved by the temporary interruption of the blood flow to the muscle itself. The chemical protection of ischemic myocardium, put simply as heart muscle deprived of oxygen, became an industry in itself. And as the techniques improved, the operations themselves became longer and more complicated – but increasingly safe.

Because progress was predicated upon applied science and evolving technology, the United States was the place to learn about them. Money mattered, details mattered and Bentall knew that the best surgical scientist in the world was John Webster Kirklin. Kirklin didn't suffer fools gladly. In fact, fools didn't last five minutes in his department. Lord Brock was said to give 'the impression of perpetual disappointment at the unattainability of universal perfection'. Kirklin refused to accept that perfection wasn't attainable. On the contrary, he insisted upon it – and that was hard to live with.

It was in September 1966 – on the same day that I started at medical school in London – that Kirklin relocated from the Mayo Clinic to Birmingham, Alabama. By the time I arrived there fifteen years later, the University of Alabama was a magnet for ambitious young cardiac surgeons from all over the world. Other centres such as the Texas Heart Institute and the Cleveland Clinic might have had greater patient throughput, but none could rival Kirklin's group for its scientific approach and academic output. My task was to assimilate that knowledge and energy, then bring it back to the NHS. If I couldn't make a name for myself in this environment, I might as well pack up and go home.

Those who had already visited Kirklin described him as an ascetic and exacting individual who strove to be the best in every aspect of the profession. He was a difficult and often intimidating man who surrounded himself with an outstanding team. 'Be under no illusion,' they told me, 'Kirklin is the boss. Cross him and you'll be out within the hour.' He held supreme power at the University of Alabama School of Medicine and, indeed, over the whole of the specialty in the US. There were good reasons for that, and Professor Bentall was absolutely right: I would be afforded no leeway here. For the first time in my career I'd need to conform, however contrary that was to my instincts.

Kirklin's legacy will always be his success in pursuit of direct vision open heart surgery with the heart–lung machine at the Mayo Clinic. This goal had initially been sought by a young Philadelphia surgeon called John Gibbon. Gibbon had been profoundly affected by watching a new mother die miserably with pulmonary embolus, a blood clot in her lungs. He set out to develop an artificial lung working in conjunction with a blood pump; this might have kept the woman alive and enabled surgeons to remove the obstruction. His complex circuit of pipes with a gas-exchange mechanism evolved into the heart–lung machine, which allowed a patient's heart to be stopped, opened and repaired under direct vision.

Yet it was not Gibbon himself who gained the ultimate prize of initiating a reliable operative technique. The first child he operated upon to close a hole in the heart died because the diagnosis was wrong, but soon afterwards on

6 May 1953 came the breakthrough the world had been waiting for. Gibbon operated on an eighteen-year-old girl and succeeded in closing an atrial septal defect. But when he attempted to repeat the operation on two five-year-old girls they both died. Gibbon walked away from the failure a broken man. In his misery and disappointment, the significance of that one success was lost on him. He lacked the resilience to recover from the girls' deaths and simply didn't possess the requisite traits to succeed as a cardiac surgeon. Uncertainty, modesty and self-doubt just don't cut the mustard.

In stark contrast, Kirklin felt that the heart–lung machine would enable the repair of more complex heart defects, so he embarked on building a 'modified Gibbon' machine in the laboratory at Mayo. On his first cardio-pulmonary bypass operation in March 1955, a child underwent closure of an atrial septal defect and survived. At this point, many of Kirklin's critics at Mayo were unconvinced by the laboratory and clinical progress. The American Heart Association and the National Institutes of Health had stopped funding further projects with heart–lung machines because they considered the problems generated by the interaction of the patient's blood with the foreign surfaces of the machine to be insurmountable.

Then in the spring of 1954 came the astonishing news that Walton Lillehei had connected the blood vessels of a baby to his father's circulation to enable him to repair a hole in the baby's heart. After this, Kirklin's critics suggested that too much money and effort had already been wasted on a blind alley. But they were wrong. When Kirklin's improved bypass circuit was used in the operating theatre, twenty-four of the first forty open heart surgery patients survived.

Kirklin undoubtedly succeeded because of his persistence and scientific approach. Even when I was with him, every operation was carefully recorded then analysed, and the information was used to assist decision-making on other patients. As he wrote:

> Academic surgery is the fusion of clinical surgery,
> research, teaching and administration. Those who
> have experienced only one of these components
> cannot understand the whole.

He instilled this principle is us trainees, and those who could not aspire to it found him very intimidating.

With more widespread adoption of cardiopulmonary bypass, it became apparent that the contact between the patient's blood and the synthetic materials within the extracorporeal circuit caused a pseudo-allergic reaction that would be referred to as the 'post-perfusion syndrome'. This sinister and sometimes fatal problem was never experienced by Lillehei's cross-circulation patients because their blood remained within a biological circuit. Some bypass patients developed fever lasting several days, with stiff, waterlogged lungs, bleeding tendencies and kidney failure. While the syndrome was often inconsequential after most straightforward adult bypasses, the more vulnerable patients, including small children or the very sick and elderly, would require prolonged periods on the ventilator, blood transfusions or kidney dialysis to survive. The longer the time spent on the bypass machine, the more likely were these complications to occur. Sometimes they resulted in the patient's death despite an effective heart repair, obviously a great disappointment to the surgeons.

At the time the heart–lung machine consisted of plastic pipes, a simple roller pump, a complex blood oxygenator and reservoir, then a suction system, all of which required priming with around two litres of anticoagulated blood containing the chemical citrate. It used to be thought that blood-type incompatibility or biochemical disturbances caused by drugs were responsible for the post-perfusion syndrome, but the problem persisted even when whole blood was replaced by other priming fluids such as dextrose or salt solution. Then a heat exchanger was included in the circuit to enable whole-body cooling. Cooling permitted a reduction in flow rates on the machine, which many thought would reduce blood damage. But this still did not prevent fever or lung and kidney damage, and the bleeding tendencies persisted.

On my first day in Alabama I found myself wandering around the hospital corridors completely lost. When I first set eyes on the great man he was surrounded by a group of grim-faced residents. By then, Kirklin was sixty-four and easily recognisable from pictures I had seen in cardiac surgical journals. He was slightly built, around 5 foot 10 inches tall and grey-haired, but it was the heavy, dark-rimmed glasses that immediately gave him away. He wore a freshly starched white lab coat with his name embroidered on it, although I was too far away to read this at the time. All I could see was a face that looked like thunder. He was angry, while his audience looked anxious and crestfallen. Had one of his patients died? No. It was just that the night team had failed to call him about a significant complication. A stroke.

Life was tough for those guys. Each resident was on call alternate nights and lucky to escape the hospital before 7 pm the following evening. And I discovered the hard way that you always had to be clean-shaven before the boss turned up in the morning. He did not tolerate sloppy or tired, even though the residents were perpetually exhausted. It was all part of the training.

As I drew closer to the group I could overhear the conversation. Kirklin wanted to know why a new resident had used a particular drug to slow a rapid heart rate. Having recently joined the service, the young man was not up to speed with the boss's strictly regimented protocols for post-operative care. He responded to the onslaught by saying that he had called Kirklin the previous night and he'd told him to use the drug.

'I don't remember that,' Kirklin replied, steam billowing out of his ears. 'I must have been sleeping. Don't you ever take an order from me again while I'm asleep.'

As I strode past the gathering, the boss concluded his tirade and turned to abandon the wobbly residents. My eyes met his, and I froze in his steely gaze.

'You're Westaby, aren't you? I've seen your picture. I was expecting you last week.'

This was a testing remark deliberately aimed at putting me on the back foot. I simply said in my best English accent, 'No sir, you are mistaken. Last week was Christmas.'

The chief resident, who'd remained at his shoulder, looked at the ceiling and rolled his eyes, anticipating a thunderbolt. Instead a broad grin broke through and Kirklin's tired eyes wrinkled behind his horn-rimmed spectacles. Englishman had contradicted the living legend and scored a touchdown in the process.

'I've been told you are difficult,' he said. 'So Bentall sent you to reform school. Come along to the office.'

Eugene 'Gene' Blackstone was there waiting for him. Blackstone had trained as a surgeon at the university but then moved over into full-time cardiovascular research. His role was to analyse the departments' data output and use it to shape day-to-day clinical practice. Some referred to Blackstone as Kirklin's auxiliary brain, and even Kirklin acknowledged him as a genius.

My own lowly title was 'international clinical fellow'. There were always several of us there at a time and we came right at the bottom of the pecking order, lab rats who helped in the operating room. But that was OK. Just to be there was special. Everyone had to start from the first rung in this environment, and we all hoped to be involved in some great research project, a ground-breaking endeavour where we could publish important papers with our names alongside the master, Kirklin, and the wizard, Blackstone. We all saw this as the ticket to success back in our own countries.

Kirklin opened by inviting me to talk about myself. Apparently the phrase 'outstanding technical surgeon but a nightmare to work with' had appeared in my references. Although I was more than content to hear that, Kirklin quite reasonably wondered what I had done to warrant the second part of the description. Was I one of those bullish public schoolboy types from Eton or Harrow? I soon disabused him of that notion. I told him about growing up in the north of England in a steel town just like Birmingham, Alabama, then watching my grandfather die from heart failure when nothing could be done to help him. I mentioned that I had worked in the steelworks and as a hospital porter to support myself through medical school. Not that any of this made me difficult – I blamed all that on the head injury. This struck a chord with Kirklin, who was an American football fan. He was intrigued that rugby was just as violent but we didn't wear helmets.

The fact that I managed to hold their attention for twenty minutes was very satisfying. It was an animated exchange and I repeatedly made them laugh. This impromptu meeting was like winning the lottery. A list of new projects had been drawn up for the year but the formal meeting to allocate the research would be later that week.

While Kirklin caught up with his secretary, Blackstone engaged with me directly. 'I've read your curriculum vitae,' he said. 'You have a degree in biochemistry. I think you can help us with something.'

Jet lagged, I smiled at him but my spirits sank. I didn't want to do fucking biochemistry. I was there to operate and show them what I was made of. So I said nothing.

Then Kirklin returned. 'I want you to work with my son on a project,' he said. 'Jim has just joined us as chief resident from Boston.'

Then I started to listen. If the boss wanted his own son involved it had to be important. As he left the office for the operating room his departing remark to me was, 'Come and join me when Gene has explained everything.'

I'd been accepted into the fold. But no more bullshit. I would never get away with it. For once I had to be a team player, not the prima donna.

The schedule in the unit was unrelenting. The residents' morning rounds began at 5 am and Kirklin was called at precisely 6 o'clock with a progress report. A minute too soon and he would put the phone down on you; a minute too late and you were in trouble when he arrived in the hospital. Surgery began after breakfast at 7 o'clock and often went on well into the evening. Morbidity and mortality were simply unacceptable, particularly through human error. Then there were the evening rounds. Full departmental academic meetings where research updates were presented took place on both Wednesday and Saturday mornings at 8 o'clock. Topic presentations or journal reviews had to be flawless. On Sunday morning at 7 o'clock Kirklin and Blackstone held academic business meetings to review progress in the various research projects and finalise scientific manuscripts for publication. Kirklin usually went riding on Sunday afternoons, while Blackstone went to church.

When the residents foolishly dared to complain of sleep deprivation following long nights in intensive care, Kirklin replaced them with clinical nurse practitioners. For the fellows like me, laboratory research would alternate with operating theatre sessions. Patient follow-up for published papers had to be exhaustive, complete with telephone calls to the coroner's office, prisons and overseas embassies until all patients had been located. One fellow working alongside me spent two years following up 5,000 coronary bypass patients to produce one single manuscript. That was the Kirklin work ethic.

The system I had to adapt to was all about perfection – the best outcomes, the lowest death rates. In the mid-1960s the surgical mortality rate for blue babies with a condition called tetralogy of Fallot exceeded 50 per cent. By 1970 in Birmingham it was 8 per cent. Come 1981, Kirklin's exacting protocols and meticulous surgery meant that any death was considered a disaster. Children simply no longer died from technical errors, and those who experienced life-threatening problems usually did so because of their exposure to the heart–lung machine. There was therefore an ongoing battle against the post-perfusion syndrome and it was time to drill down to the cause. This was to be my research. I had the appropriate background to dig deep and discover the biochemical triggers for these damaging effects. Right place, right time, right project.

So what was already known? With certainty, it was the contact between the patient's own blood and the myriad of plastics and metals in the bypass circuit that initiated the reaction. Most tissues of the body seemed to be affected by it, and the full-blown syndrome was always accompanied by a swinging temperature that persisted for two or three days, together with a rise in white blood cell count. These were also the features of a blood-borne infection or septicaemia. So my hypothesis was that we were investigating whole-body inflammation, in contrast to the local inflammatory response that occurs in pneumonia, appendicitis or a boil.

When the syndrome proved fatal, the autopsy findings often supported that generalised inflammatory concept. Just as occurred with an infected cut, fluid – known as oedema – leaked into the tissues, causing them to swell. In the lungs this caused laboured breathing, low blood-oxygen levels and sometimes frank bleeding into the bronchial tubes. Similar swelling in the brain caused what was known as post-pump delirium – agitation and confusion, making the patient difficult to control. Then kidney function would deteriorate, causing even more fluid to be held in the body. The whole process tended to be self-limiting and disappeared within a week, but the frail or sicker patients did not survive it.

To improve our clinical response to the syndrome we needed to know its cause. Gene Blackstone had made it clear that there were substantial resources to support the project and that I would be expected to work out what could be done about it. As the new chief resident, Jim Kirklin would help with patient studies, and I even had laboratory technicians assigned to assist me. They were giving me every opportunity to change cardiac surgery.

I started the detective work by devouring the literature on inflammation. What was it that stimulated white blood cells to come together and attack bacteria or foreign bodies such as splinters in the skin? What caused infected tissues to accumulate fluid and weep serum? Tipped off by Blackstone, I read that kidney dialysis patients suffered lung problems too. The dialysis and heart–lung machines had much in common – plastic tubing and synthetic membranes in broad contact with blood. The dialysis machine exchanges toxic chemicals, the heart–lung machine exchanges gases, but the materials at the blood–foreign surface interface were similar.

Scientists and kidney physicians at the University of Minnesota had already found some clues. They showed that a little-known chain of proteins in the blood called the complement system was activated by contact with the dialysis membrane and that toxins released by the reaction caused white blood cells to adhere to the lining of the blood vessels in the lungs. What's more, the Scripps Research Institute in San Diego had developed a chemical assay to measure the amounts of toxin circulating in the blood. I was so excited and energised by reading all this that I rushed straight from the library to Blackstone's office to inform him of my line of investigation.

Mildly amused by the eccentric Englishman, Gene swivelled around in his chair and responded in a Deep Southern drawl. 'I wondered how long it would take you to uncover that paper. Get on and call Scripps. Ask if they will take blood samples from us, then come back to me with your protocol. Have a good day!'

I suggested that we should take serial blood samples from a consecutive series of Kirklin's patients who were having operations both with and without the bypass machine. Then we would carefully record the severity of the post-perfusion syndrome by assessing brain, lung and kidney function, together with blood clotting during their recovery. The object of the exercise was to determine whether blood levels of the toxins could be linked to the degree of post-operative organ dysfunction in the patient.

It was a great project for me because I could spend all day in the operating theatre watching or assisting with the operations, then learn more about intensive care as I collected the blood samples overnight. These were the places I wanted to be, not in some boring laboratory washing test tubes, although I had my fair share of that while preparing the blood samples to be dispatched to California. It was when I was bold enough to tell Kirklin that I wanted to scrub in with the surgery, not just to watch, that another technician was allocated to work with me. This was my reward for staying in the hospital around the clock and not being as troublesome as Bentall had predicted.

Having Jack assigned to work with me brought further opportunities and suggested an obvious plan. If the blood–foreign surface interaction was the trigger, it would be great to find out which of the many synthetic materials were problematic and whether the temperature within the bypass circuit made a difference. Going off piste again, I set up my own little biochemistry lab and, with Jack's help, spirited away expensive bypass equipment from the perfusionists' storeroom. We broke down the various polymers and plastic tubes into pieces small enough to fit into a test tube, then incubated them with fresh human blood. We just paid students for an armful, no big deal in those days.

I eventually collected samples from 116 patients on cardiopulmonary bypass and from a dozen who'd had shunt operations or vascular repairs without the machine. None of the non-bypass operations showed a rise in toxin levels, telling us that neither the anaesthetic nor the surgery itself triggered a significant inflammatory reaction. Now the exciting bit – all the cardiopulmonary bypass patients had shedloads of toxins released in their blood, and the longer the patient remained on the heart–lung machine, the higher the levels rose. Moreover, the higher the level of toxins, the more likely the patient was to suffer lung, kidney and brain dysfunction afterwards. Even post-operative heart failure seemed to be related to high levels of toxin release. Eleven of the bypass patients died, and there was a close correlation between elevated toxin levels and risk of death.

Huge amounts of data were generated during these experiments. Consequently, it took weeks of detailed analysis by Gene Blackstone to unravel the findings. In essence, we had finally identified the mechanism of the post-perfusion syndrome. The toxins released by blood–foreign surface interaction stuck to the patient's white blood cell membranes, causing them to aggregate and initiate inflammation in the vital organs. Using strategically placed catheters in the operating theatre, I showed that virtually half of the body's circulating white blood cells became trapped in the patient's lungs at the end of cardiopulmonary bypass when we allowed blood to flow back into them again. It was oxygen free radicals and protein digestive enzymes released from the trapped white cells that damaged the delicate tissue membranes. I remember presenting these extraordinary findings to the research meeting and the stunned silence they caused. Silence – followed by great excitement. But what was the point of discovering all this if nothing could be done about it? That's where my covert efforts in the laboratory bore fruit.

The hours in the operating theatre were long, then I would join Jack in the laboratory to work on the synthetic materials. What we heard from Scripps was a complete revelation. Medical-grade nylon, which was widely approved for use in dialysis and heart–lung machines, strongly activated the complement system. Other materials did too, but to a lesser degree. Before we demonstrated this, nylon's propensity to release damaging chemicals did not feature in any assessment of biocompatibility. I could now see the way forward. We could clearly make a difference. I explained my tinkering in the background to Gene Blackstone and then to Kirklin. The results from our materials testing were shown to the companies who manufactured the oxygenators and blood reservoirs for the bypass machines. Presented with the evidence, they worked a way to remove the nylon and substitute more blood-compatible materials. Then we waited to see whether this would make a difference.

With a successful project under my belt, I spent more and more time scrubbing in with the surgeons. Kirklin was regimented and fastidious. He took his time and did nothing without a good reason. Every move was based on measurement, algorithms and protocol. The incision had to be a certain length, the patch a certain diameter, the valve a particular size, all carefully correlated with the patient's body weight. Nothing was ever left to chance, and he was easily irritated when onlookers asked too many questions during a case. Yet he seemed to take a shine to the eccentric Englishman, and wrote kind and encouraging letters when I was back in London.

In the adjacent theatre was Al Pacifico, the complete antithesis to Kirklin and the swiftest and most spontaneous surgeon I'd ever watched. By 1981 it was Pacifico who was operating on the most complex congenital heart disease cases, the twisted, contorted hearts full of holes or obstructed ventricles. Everything he did looked straightforward, effortless and second nature. I would step back from the operating table and write down or draw every critical step. This became my 'play book' of congenital heart surgery, an invaluable resource when I inaugurated my own paediatric programme in Oxford.

Often there would be just Pacifico, with me across the table and a physician's assistant at my side. Although physician assistants, universally known as PAs, were not doctors, they were trained to remove leg veins for coronary bypass operations, to open and close chests, and to assist the surgeon with parts of other operations. Experienced PAs did these things just as well as the surgical residents; in turn, their presence eventually enabled the residents to cover the intensive care unit and post-operative wards, making their long days manageable. A nurse anaesthetist, again without medical training, would primarily look after an adult case, while a medically qualified anaesthesiologist would supervise two or three operating rooms.

I was intrigued by this approach, but I doubted whether operating PAs or nurse anaesthetists could ever be sanctioned in the NHS. The British medical profession was far too arrogant and self-interested to acknowledge that any aspect of their work could be undertaken without the statutory six years at medical school. In reality, PAs were trained in half that time and were far more cost-effective. I remembered thinking that I would do this when I got a consultant job back home. Bugger the establishment.

We soon found that oxygenators and circuits without nylon were indeed making a difference – patients spent less time on the ventilator and in the intensive care unit because their lungs were better, and fewer died. In addition, there was a decrease in post-operative blood transfusion and the need for kidney dialysis fell away. This had massive economic implications and that fundamental piece of research saved many thousands of lives, indeed infinitely more than I saved over my whole surgical career. I started to get invitations to lecture throughout North America, and Blackstone was happy for me to do this. The name Westaby became known to the great and the good of US cardiac surgery, as well as those in the cardiovascular industry.

In the midst of this success I heard that Dr Cooley had implanted a total artificial heart in Houston, only the second ever attempted. It was a Friday morning. Audaciously, that same evening I set out for Houston on the 'red eye', determined to meet the great man and see the remarkable technology for myself. I felt like one of the wise men making my way to Bethlehem to meet the baby Jesus. Like me, Dr Cooley had trained at the Brompton, so I had an opening gambit. I accosted him out of the blue at 6.30 am at the entrance of St Luke's Hospital and was kindly received. He took me to see the patient in their 120-bed intensive care unit and later that night I was called back to watch the heart transplant. The artificial heart was rubbish, the overall experience sensational. This visit began my long association with the Texas Heart Institute and mechanical circulatory support.

For me, Birmingham had worked its magic. I had seen and participated in so much that I now felt like a real cardiac surgeon. What's more, I was given the chance to remain in the States – the highly disciplined environment had smoothed away my rough edges and my technical skills were considered to be worth keeping. But that could never happen. I had a daughter back home and I had to return.

6

joy

9 PM, CHRISTMAS 1985. I was slumped on an uncomfortable wooden bench in the accident department of St Thomas' – Florence Nightingale's famous hospital opposite the Palace of Westminster – in the company of bandaged heads, bleeding noses and puking drunks. In reality they were more mental health problems than actual emergencies. 'Joy to the World' played incongruously over the intercom and for this tramp it was the perfect place to spend the evening.

As the night staff reluctantly dribbled in, the late shift were desperate to get home, so none of them were at all interested in a sad character in a tatty Santa Claus outfit slouching by a dying tree whose lights had fused. Sister in charge was gliding in and out of the waiting area, doing her best to raise spirits. At St Thomas', nursing sisters still looked the part. This Christmas angel was tall, slim and elegant in a navy spotted dress and sheer black tights. With her small waist and a silver belt buckle, her jet-black hair framed between a starched white collar and a formal cap adorned with mistletoe, this woman – equally

renowned in body and mind – was known throughout St
Thomas' as 'Sister Beautiful'. Doctors, ambulance men
and police fawned round her, trying to pick their moment,
hoping to take advantage of that seasonal invitation on
her cap – a kiss from an angel, just for that one night of
the year, a consolation for having to work on Christmas
Day.

She glanced across the room at me and asked one of the
staff nurses to find out what Santa Claus needed. Had I
just come in to escape the cold night? If so, they should
give me hot tea and some cake that she had brought in
herself for her frequent flyers, the vagrants and destitute
of south London. She didn't recognise me behind the
beard. She wasn't meant to.

Outside, an ambulance pulled up on the frosty gantry,
sounding its siren by the main entrance. Anticipating trouble, Sister Beautiful and the duty casualty officer headed
towards the swing doors. It was a heart attack patient
already in shock. As the paramedics lowered the trolley to
the pavement, the blip, blip, blip of the monitor ceased and
the random spikey waves of ventricular fibrillation triggered an alarm. They moved swiftly to the resuscitation
room through the piped strains of 'Silent Night', and with
a sense of urgency Sister climbed onto the trolley, strad-
dled the man's waist and began pumping frantically on his
chest. She shouted to the mesmerised casualty officer to
run ahead and charge the defibrillator. 'All is calm' and
'sleep in heavenly peace' seemed lost in the moment.

This cardiac surgeon could only watch anonymously in
admiration, unable to do anything to help. I didn't belong

there. Sister Beautiful had the presence of mind to instruct the night staff to look after the man's wife, then, still pounding away, she disappeared from sight. I glanced across the waiting room to the crib in the corner. There were angels there too. With a flurry of activity the cardiac resuscitation team arrived from the wards and piled in behind this extraordinary woman. Then the door closed behind them.

I had been Santa Claus for the Hammersmith Hospital children's ward early that morning. Only really sick kids stay in for Christmas and some of them had cancer. Emaciated, anaemic and bald from chemotherapy, they had swung their bony little legs out of their beds, waiting for me to arrive with their present. Their loving parents propped them up and tried to divert their minds from the exhaustion and misery of it all, if only for a few minutes. There were smiles and a few tears, not least from Santa himself. I knew it could be their last time. Then, with a sense of relief and a huge sack of my own daughter's presents on the back seat of the car, I headed for the North Circular road and the A10 to Cambridge. Gemma was seven now and I made the same journey each year. It was always a happy day, until I had to leave. Watching her wave me goodbye on the doorstep cracked me up every time, and I'd weep pitifully all the way back to London. Yet there was no one to blame but myself.

Although I spoke with her every single day, I was obsessed by the fact that I had deprived her of a normal childhood. A huge surgical ego was one thing, but I had little self-respect, seeing myself as a shit parent with no moral compass who worked perpetually. The more I did, the less my aging bosses had to do – and that suited them.

Sarah – Sister Beautiful – was gone for an hour. Eventually she emerged from the resus room looking dishevelled and dejected, her white cap and collar long gone, her tights laddered and the top buttons of her dress open. Performing cardiac massage for a prolonged period is equivalent to a vigorous workout at the gym. Beads of sweat were rolling from her neck and disappearing down the valley between her breasts. The medical students stared at her shamelessly as she disappeared into the relatives' room, where the wail of despair from the disconsolate wife told most of the story. Meanwhile the tape had gone full circle and the waiting room was treated once more to 'Joy to the World'.

It was close to 11 pm and the bossy night sister was making strenuous efforts to clear the department of the alcoholics and walking wounded. The charade was over. I had spied on my lover for long enough, but it had been worth it. I hadn't watched Sarah do what she did best since Cambridge, where she had looked after my rugby injuries – fractured jaw, torn scalp, cracked ribs, none of which stopped me getting straight back to the operating theatre.

Despite being two hours beyond the end of her shift, she still had one last task. The anguished wife wanted to see the man with whom she had shared her life one last time before that plaque ruptured in his main coronary artery and acute heart failure killed him. I might have rushed him onto a heart–lung machine and bypassed the blockage, but not here in St Thomas'. This was Sarah's hospital, not mine. The on-call cardiac surgeons were miles away at home, not hanging around for some excitement.

When Sarah finally emerged from that room of death, Santa was standing right outside so she couldn't miss me. She looked pale and stressed. It had been eleven hours of verbal abuse, being spat at, then mauled by drunks and boisterous junior doctors who were queuing to give her a ride home because her anticipated lift had not turned up. Or so it had seemed. Now she had to cope with an emotional car crash of a lover before coming back for 8 o'clock the following morning.

Both of us needed to wind down and talk, and Westminster Bridge at midnight was made for that. We leaned over the parapet and stared down into the ice-cold Thames, me in Santa's coat, Sarah in her black nurse's cape, as Big Ben commenced its countdown to midnight. By now it was an unusually silent night, everyone at home in bed apart from the human flotsam and jetsam that was still drifting into the accident department. Same at the Hammersmith, same at Charing Cross, same everywhere. Sarah had seen three deaths that shift – the cardiac man, and two lonely young suicides for whom Christmas had become unbearable. She was upset about the girl in particular, a sixteen-year-old thrown out by her family for getting pregnant. She had sought an abortion but couldn't afford it, so had leapt from a railway bridge. And when it didn't seem that I was there at the end of her shift, Sister

Beautiful had thought the worst about me too. One way or another.

Christmas 1987. I was three months into my consultant post in Oxford, excited to have been taken on by the world's foremost academic brand to set up a new cardio-thoracic centre. For anyone who lacked my disinhibited brain, starting out single-handed as a heart surgeon would have been a daunting prospect, with no one to call upon for help or advice and no senior colleagues with whom to discuss difficult cases. But that was exactly what I loved about it, as it meant that I could stand on my own two feet. Professionally I was ruthlessly ambitious and supremely confident, and I wanted to do things differently.

The various factions in Oxford all had differing requirements – the adult cardiologists wanted an accomplished coronary artery and valve surgeon; the chest physicians insisted that lung surgery should be done by an experienced thoracic surgeon; the paediatric cardiologists were hoping for someone who could develop a congenital heart programme for them. The first surgeon in was expected to set up the whole service. In reality it was complete madness, but I revelled in the challenge.

In the background I had the most caring and selfless woman I knew, paddling hard to keep me afloat. Although Sarah was thirty-eight weeks pregnant, she still insisted that I drive to Cambridge to spend the day with Gemma and her mum. As New Year came then passed, so did Sarah's due date; but I was so absorbed in my own personal indispensability that our impending childbirth barely impacted on me. Nothing seemed more exciting than operating on hearts, which says something about my cerebral cortex at the time. Still bruised, I guess. Sarah was trying to educate me in the ways of empathy, but I had some distance to go.

20 January 1988, now ten days overdue. The midwife started talking about induction. Mark was a good-sized baby but his head was still not engaged (no change there, then!). But with a good, steady foetal heart rate there were no real concerns and Sarah wanted to let nature take its course.

In my parallel world things were about to kick off. I was on the wards, conducting an early morning round before theatre. Today there were just boring coronary bypasses on the operating list, patients who had waited months for surgery in London hospitals before being clawed back for the new surgeon to operate on. Unexpectedly I received a call from the duty cardiology registrar. His boss Dr Gribben, a dour Scotsman, had requested an urgent opinion on a sick patient before I committed myself to the operating theatre for the whole day.

This was an unfortunate twenty-two-year-old woman with Down's syndrome, who had come in with an infection in her blood stream – sepsis, as we call it. I could have made up the rest of the story without asking. As with many Down's children, Megan had undergone repair of a complete atrioventricular canal defect in infancy – literally a void at the centre of the heart, with valves that had not formed properly. The reconstructed mitral valve had always leaked, and now it was infected with the aggressive *Staphylococcus aureus* bacterium. Endocarditis is the medical term for this, and it would undoubtedly progress rapidly and prove fatal. She would certainly need a mitral valve replacement as soon as possible.

My initial response was that we should get on and do it that same day. As I've mentioned, I'd had an affinity for these affectionate, genetically disadvantaged kids since they were denied corrective operations at the Brompton 'because it wasn't worth it'. They were said not to fare as well as normal children with congenital heart disease, but that simply wasn't true. I was destined to correct more than two hundred atrioventricular canal defects in Oxford, with a vanishingly low mortality rate. But there was more to come. Dr Gribben came along himself and, looking me straight in the eye, said that there was something else I needed to know. It transpired that the parents, who had adopted Megan from an orphanage, were Jehovah's Witnesses and that there was no way they would accept a blood transfusion.

These few words added a new dimension of agonising complexity to the case, and I could tell that Gribben expected me to flatly turn her down at this point. First, unlike non-cardiac surgery, the heart–lung machine dilutes the circulation with its priming fluid. Then reoperations always bleed more. Finally, patients with sepsis have abnormal coagulation and may bleed heavily, so without blood they are likely to die. Heart surgery only became possible after the emergence of both blood transfusion and antibiotics during the Second World War. But in 1945 the governing body of Jehovah's Witnesses introduced the blood ban based on a strict literal interpretation of the Bible. Interestingly, Jehovah's Witnesses celebrate neither Christmas nor birthdays, are politically neutral, do not enlist in the military nor salute flags. I always accepted them for surgery, but it was a challenge to get them through. These days, with death rates thrust into the public arena, many of my colleagues will not take the chance.

Although Megan was twenty-two, I did not feel that she had sufficient understanding of her plight either to consent to the operation or consciously reject transfused blood if her life were threatened. So it was down to her adoptive parents to make decisions on her behalf. Sure enough they produced a legally binding 'advanced directive' prohibiting a blood transfusion. I had long since learned to avoid unnecessary polarisation and potential conflict over religious beliefs, and would never have confronted them by saying that their daughter was going to die without blood or that I wasn't prepared to operate unless I could transfuse her. To be honest, blood transfusion is undesirable for many reasons and inherently increases surgical mortality. I would avoid it myself unless I was otherwise doomed. Yet in my own mind I was not going to let this girl bleed to death. She had been born with enough bad luck without me terminating her life needlessly.

The parents took the position that they would only sign the consent form if the anaesthetist, the intensive care doctors and I promised that we would not use blood. We were also asked not to pursue a court order to do so. So what was acceptable to them? I explained that there was a new machine called a cell saver that would scavenge spilled blood and give it back to Megan. Blood lost into the wound is suctioned, centrifuged and washed, then mixed with an anticoagulant before being put back into the patient via a filter. The filter removes bacteria and white blood cells, making it an important tool in the treatment of sepsis. That was not so different from the heart–lung machine, whose tubing we primed with clear fluid. The cell saver was acceptable because it was her own blood circulating continuously, and Jehovah's Witnesses were usually content with that, as with kidney dialysis. They both nodded in agreement. I had a couple of other tricks up my sleeve that I did not want to discuss at this stage, so we agreed to proceed on their terms.

Clearly I was sticking my neck out with this case. I had only been operating in Oxford for three months and had encountered a particular arrogance that was hard to justify, something along the lines of 'We are Oxford, so we must be good.' It was curiously different from Addenbrooke's in Cambridge; indeed with his usual pragmatism Roy Calne had already warned me about what to expect. I was only allowed to use eight beds on a general surgical ward, then after surgery the patients had to go to the general intensive care unit shared by trauma, acute medicine, obstetrics and other surgical specialties. As a result I needed to fight for a bed for practically every case.

Then it transpired that good old Theatre 5 was completely unsuitable for cardiac surgery, much more so than I had initially realised. There was no piped oxygen into the room and its single heart–lung machine belonged in a museum. Alarms would sound and Ted, my only perfusionist, would jump up, disconnect the empty oxygen cylinder and dash outside for a replacement. A perfusionist must never leave his machine during a case, but Ted left during every single one. He had no alternative in his efforts to keep us afloat.

Soon after my arrival there was a catastrophic failure of the antique machine's heater–cooler system at the beginning of an operation. We needed to cool then rewarm the patient to repair her heart, but we'd lost our ability to do so. Before we could attach the unsuspecting woman to the circuit, Ted ran out of theatre and returned with a bucket and a bowl. He filled the bucket with tap water and ice for cooling, then prior to rewarming he fetched a kettle of warm water for the bowl. The bypass tubing with the blood flowing through it was simply flipped from bucket to bowl when I gave the order to rewarm. This tableau was more suited to a Monty Python film than a major teaching hospital, but I soon learned that it had been going on like this for years.

Then the scrub sink blocked. The overhead lights had a life of their own, so I would perpetually be desterilising myself when adjusting their position. Next, sewage leaked through the ceiling from the toilets above. Eventually I decided to call the long-suffering hospital manager Mr Stapleton when anything went wrong. I would stamp my foot and tell Sister Linda, 'Send for Mr Stapleton.' More often than not he would actually appear in his suit at the door of Theatre 5 and say, 'What is it now, Westaby?' Without shifting my gaze from the heart, I would bellow that it was the bloody this or the bloody that, while the anaesthetist Tony Fisher would duck behind the anaesthetic screen giggling to himself. But in the end we didn't lose anyone. Against all odds, my first hundred patients in Oxford all survived.

Now came the tricky bit. We obviously didn't have the cell saver machine I needed to attempt a reoperation on a Jehovah's Witness, so I frantically set about trying to locate the company representative to persuade him to lend us one. The earliest this could happen was the following day, late in the morning. That would give us twenty-four hours to soak Megan in high-dose antibiotics, but I insisted that in the meantime she should be carefully observed in the intensive care unit. I had an ulterior motive for this – at least she would be guaranteed a bed after the surgery, and we couldn't wait any longer. I also insisted that she be given a hormone called erythropoietin – the infamous EPO of professional cycling – which boosts red blood cell formation in the bone marrow. This, together with high-dose iron, vitamin B12 and folic acid, would help her make up her haemoglobin levels in the days and weeks after surgery, when I expected her to be severely anaemic. Tomorrow I would also give her an agent called aprotinin, which I had personally, albeit inadvertently, found to assist blood clotting in patients on cardiopulmonary bypass. Another landmark advance for the specialty.

Halfway through the first coronary bypass that morning, Tony the anaesthetist leaned over the screen and whispered something to me. I was concentrating on sewing a vein to a tiny but critical coronary artery and didn't hear, so I asked him to repeat what he'd just said. This time the whole operating theatre heard.

'We've just had a call to say your wife is having contractions and there is no one who can drive her to the hospital.'

My reply – 'Can't she still drive herself?' – was insensitive, to say the least.

In unison the nursing staff groaned. *Nul points* for that suggestion.

I touted the next option – 'Tell her to call for a taxi.' What else could I say? I was operating on someone's heart, with another hugely difficult case in waiting.

As it was, Sarah called her midwife, who went to the house, stuck in a fist and said, 'You're not dilating yet. Better to stay here for now. The hospital will only send you home.'

It might sound like callous disregard for me to have carried on operating all day, but there was no one else to take over. What's more, I considered childbirth to be a natural physiological event, not something to go 'gaga-gooey' about, then turn it into some sort of cataclysmic phenomenon, as normal people do. When I'd been a medical student I had delivered my allocated two dozen babies at Neasden Maternity Hospital in north London, although I found the repair of ragged perineal tears more compelling than catching the greasy neonate before it slipped out onto the floor. Having said that, I was always very sympathetic to the mothers. I wouldn't want to push a melon out of my arse, let alone a whole baby. But however much fussing and fawning I might have done for Sarah, it wouldn't have made the following few hours any more comfortable for her, so I was better employed plumbing hearts.

That's what I tried to persuade myself, at least. But it wasn't the whole story, and I think Sarah knew the truth of the matter – that I wasn't there with my first wife Jane when Gemma was born. My own dear mother was around to help, but I was miles away and my conscience was considerably troubled about that. So this was a difficult time for me, although Sarah was such a bloody saint that she was mentally adjusted to go it alone. Gradually she was chipping away at my neuroses without arguments or conflict, just unwavering support. She realised I had massive professional challenges ahead but was willing me to succeed in Oxford, whatever it took. What's more, people used to think I must be a good guy for someone that special to have married me.

When I finally got back home in the evening, Sarah's contractions were becoming more intense and painful. Mark had decided it was time to escape. I prepared a warm bath for her but as she clambered out her waters broke, gushing amniotic fluid all over the bathroom floor. I had absolutely no recollection of those student deliveries yet suspected that breaching of the dam was a good reason to seek help from someone who knew what they were doing. We arrived at the John Radcliffe maternity unit at 10.30 pm and went directly to the prenatal ward.

As always, they were busy. Once more they wanted to gauge the degree of cervical dilation before committing Sarah to a bed. Again the lad's head wasn't engaged. Delivery would not be any time soon.

To the surprise of the ward sister, my response was stern and to the point. 'Please take good care of them both. I have two heart operations tomorrow and need to get some sleep. I'll come back at around 6.30 in the morning.'

Stoical saintly Sarah was fine with that. Maternity sister looked as if she had just pissed her pants. So this was the new heart surgeon everyone was talking about.

The only phone call overnight was from the intensive care unit to bleat that they were worried about Megan. She was febrile, her blood pressure was bumping along the bottom at around 90/60 and there was precious little urine in the bag.

I was a bit direct with the duty registrar, along the lines of, 'The cell saver arrives tomorrow. If you want to operate on her without it, get the fuck on with it. Otherwise get your own consultant to come in and help.'

Working single-handed, on call every night and every weekend for months on end, is wearing. I was perpetually exhausted and sleep deprived. Not that anyone could give a shit, except my wife. I felt desperately sorry for her now. She deserved much better. In fact she'd had much better, until I screwed things up for her. I picked up the phone again and called the prenatal unit to ask about her. Essentially no change; the pain was rumbling on. That's the way it is in obstetrics. Pain is the price women pay.

27 January 1988, 6 am. It was going to be a difficult day. I was with Sarah early for a few minutes' commiseration, then hurried to intensive care at 7 o'clock with the intention of being pleasant to the young doctor I'd abused on the phone. Sarah had been pale and drawn after a night in agony. Would I have let one of my own patients suffer like that? Absolutely not. I resolved to ring her obstetrician before I began operating and tell him I wanted to see my son between cases. My cases, that is, not his. I didn't want to embark on a complex reoperation on a septic young woman while I was worrying about my own wife and child. But in the end I didn't make the call. It would have been stupid to antagonise those who were caring for her when I was so bloody useless myself. I was the passive partner in all this, not occupying my usual role of dishing out orders.

My first patient that morning had an aortic valve replacement and was safely back in intensive care by 11 am. But where the hell was the cell saver? Instead of returning to maternity to check on Sarah, I needed to make sure that everyone knew what to expect during the battle that would be Megan's operation. It was too late now for Ted to learn how to put the cell saver together, so the company representative would have to stay with us in theatre and set it all up himself. Tony needed to get on and infuse the aprotinin before I ran the saw up Megan's chest.

This was all new for Theatre 5. It all felt like we were on stage at the first night of a West End play for which we hadn't done any rehearsals, with the lead actor wanted in another part of the hospital to play a crucial supporting role. The curtain was about to go up for his leading lady, but the cad was nowhere to be seen.

I expect that was how Sarah's obstetrician and midwives must have felt about it. They were used to syco-phantic, fawning husbands who sat clinging to their wives' hands and rubbing their backs, very different from my own birth in 1948 when the father of the blue baby in the next cot couldn't even get an hour away from the steelworks.

We had chosen Sarah's obstetrician because I had oper-ated with him on a pregnant endocarditis case in which we'd performed a caesarean section then an aortic valve reoperation at the same sitting. Mother and baby both survived, but I knew of similar cases with 200 per cent mortality. I was sure he would take good care of Sarah when the time came, although I was now scrubbing up for another long operation without knowing when that would be. Secretly I hoped that the delivery would be over for Sarah by the time I emerged.

Across in the maternity suite the prolonged and painful birth process that I had hoped would be physiological was gradually evolving into pathological. Sarah was now physically and psychologically exhausted. As understand-ing as she had been of my personal demons, she was now justifiably pissed off that I wasn't around when she needed me, although the fact remained that I wouldn't have been any bloody good had I been there. Temperamentally I am not someone who can wait for things to happen and allow someone else to be in charge. Surgeons are not built that way, and being irritated and aggressive with the staff wouldn't have helped either one of us. The 'C' word had been discussed, but Sarah still wanted to avoid that if at all possible. Yet after twenty hours in labour my boy's head still wasn't engaged. He was having second thoughts about leaving his warm cocoon and the reassurance of his mother's heartbeat.

Back in Theatre 5, Megan's situation was so precarious that she was anaesthetised on the operating table, with her mother trying to keep her calm. Because of her Down's syndrome she understood little of her plight, and was terrified by the glaring lights and the cold, clinical surroundings. Her anaesthetist Mike Sinclair, with Asterix the Gaul tattooed on his arm, appreciated that a needle hovering above her might well precipitate a panic attack. So he was talking to her kindly while wafting sleepy gas over her face through a rubber mask. This was nothing to do with pity or indeed compassion. It was simply smart and engaged anaesthetics. Had the girl thrown a fit and rolled off the table, she might well have suffered a cardiac arrest and died.

I never allowed myself to empathise with someone I was about to operate on. Empathy means sharing the patient's emotions or distress and is a huge mistake for a cardiac surgeon. I never dared to imagine how it would be to lie on cold, black vinyl waiting for my blood to be drained into a machine by some psychopath. To carve open someone's chest I needed calm and clinical objectivity. Bugger empathy. Imagine being an empathetic psychiatrist or children's cancer doctor. You wouldn't last the week without suffering a breakdown.

At that moment my concern for Sarah caused me to stop scrubbing and walk to the phone in the anaesthetic room. I felt huge pangs of guilt that I was applying the same cold objectivity to my own wife. I had reverted to where I was when Gemma was born, and probably because of those very circumstances. Clearly I still hadn't shaken off my post-traumatic psychopathy. On the flip side, had my boldness abated I might have taken the sensible decision and refused to operate on Megan without blood, confronting her adopted parents with a court order and making their lives miserable. We still could give blood against their wishes, which would see them excommunicated from their church. So counterintuitively, my disinhibited approach was an act of kindness for these people. But where was I when Sister Beautiful and my own child needed me? In the fucking operating theatre, as usual.

The maternity unit phone kept ringing, but nobody answered. I tried to call Sarah's mobile, then the nurses' station – no one wanted to talk to me. Mike shouted to let me know that Megan's blood pressure was dropping, so I was obliged to get cracking on a taxing operation that could easily last six hours. It required my utmost concentration, with every millilitre of spilled blood having to be scavenged and returned to the circuit. I needed to set aside all thoughts of the maternity unit and my own anxieties for that entire time.

I heard the phone ring in the anaesthetic room about forty-five minutes into the case, when we'd already gone onto the bypass machine. A nurse soon appeared in theatre to announce that the obstetrician needed to talk with me, so I asked her to find out what he wanted while keeping my gaze fixed on the heart as it emptied out then flopped about in a meaningless way.

'He won't say. It's confidential,' came the reply, as a wave of anxiety rippled through me.

I asked Mike to ring back and see what he wanted, hoping that the obstetrician would pass on the message through a fellow consultant. Again no one answered from maternity. Mike, who had an anaesthetic senior registrar with him, said he would go across himself to find out what was happening.

'Typical cardiac surgeon,' my scrub nurse whispered. 'Sends an anaesthetist to sort out his wife's delivery.'

It would have been like an Ealing comedy had it not been so bloody worrying.

I was sewing in the artificial mitral valve when Ted chipped in. 'Steve, we seem to be getting low on volume. Have you lost any blood?'

To my knowledge we hadn't, but I asked our guest cell saver expert to put back what we had scavenged into the heart–lung machine. Ted said that this wasn't making much difference and asked me to check the pleural cavities, the space around the lungs, which are not ventilated during cardiopulmonary bypass. Sure enough, Ted was right. Around a litre of fluid had collected on the left side via a hole in the pericardium behind the heart. When we sucked that back into the circuit, things improved.

Fifteen minutes later, Mike returned.

'What news, Mike? Did you see Sarah?' I asked tentatively, not sure what to say.

'Yes, she's OK but very pissed off with you. She needs a caesarean, but they don't want to go ahead without discussing it. They're fucking scared of you.'

Our cell saver man was intrigued but bewildered by the situation. He was bold enough to suggest that I might invite a colleague to finish the operation, then even more confused to hear that I had no colleagues. The band had to keep playing even if the ship was sinking, and I was already sewing as fast as I could. Eventually Megan crept off bypass, with a shedload of vasoconstrictor drugs to combat the sepsis. But she still needed clear fluid transfusion to keep her blood pressure up, and I had to stem bleeding from the heart and wound edges before I could think about leaving.

It was 6 pm before we were ready to close Megan's chest, but her blood pressure was sagging and her plasma haemoglobin level was now critically low, so much so that I made the decision to risk lowering her body temperature with a cooling blanket to reduce tissue oxygen consumption. Red blood cells are needed to carry oxygen to the tissues, but dropping the temperature from 37°C down to 32°C would decrease oxygen consumption almost by half, around 7 per cent for each degree of cooling. The lower the temperature, however, the greater the risk of lethal heart rhythm problems. I still didn't want to ruin Megan's parents' lives by giving her blood, nor was I prepared to let her die on what I expected would be my son's birthday.

I was arranging the cooling blanket when we had another call from maternity, this time with greater urgency. They wanted me across there directly, but until Megan was safely ensconced in intensive care I was morally obliged to stay with her. My registrar Neil Moat, who would become a distinguished heart surgeon at the Brompton, went over with the message for them to get on with whatever they needed to do and that the boss would be there as soon as possible. In other words, 'You do the obstetrics, he'll do the cardiac surgery.'

At 6.30 I called Megan's parents in the relatives' room to say that the operation was over and we had not given her any blood. I told them that the recovery period would be long and difficult, and that we could not guarantee her survival. Should they reconsider the blood issue at any stage, I encouraged them to let us know, although I appreciated that this would be impossible, even with Megan at death's door. Now I had to see Sarah. She'd been in labour for twenty-six hours without me, so I wasn't expecting a warm welcome. I met Neil on his way back. He told me that Sarah was already on her way for the caesarean and urged me to go to her, leaving Megan to him.

Wearing blood-stained theatre gear, I arrived in the labour ward still secretly hoping that the job was done. The nursing sister darted from one noisy cubicle to another, doing her best to ignore me. I guess I deserved that, but it was not what I needed after a difficult day. When I was agitated enough to ask where the obstetrics theatre was, I received an ear bashing.

'Do you think your poor wife has had an easier day? She went to theatre half an hour ago. Perhaps you might like to join her.'

I dug the hole ever deeper by suggesting that Sarah would already be asleep, and I should wait to see mother and baby in the recovery room. Wrong. After many hours of pain and suffering, she had insisted on staying awake to see him arrive – no general anaesthetic, an epidural catheter instead. And because of that, she had requested that I join her if I could find the time.

The anaesthetic room was empty, but I noticed the remnants of drug vials, drips and catheters that had already been shoved into my wife. I shuffled past her discarded slippers on the trolley and peered through the crack in the theatre doors. It was the same team that I had worked with on the combined caesarean section and valve replacement, including the affable rugby-playing neonatologist Peter Hope, whose giant hands regularly performed miracles for diminutive premature babies. The empty swab rack and rattling of instruments told me that they hadn't started yet. As Sarah's anaesthetist turned to hang a bag of dextrose on the drip pole, I could see her black curls turning to follow his movements. They seemed to be chatting calmly as the overhead lights were adjusted to shine on the bump that would soon be my delivered son. This had got to be the time to go in, but there was one thing to do first – leave my phone in one of Sarah's slippers. Being called out of this operation was simply not an option.

At least my appearance was well received this time. As the door creaked open there was a collective chorus of 'He's here at last.' This was undoubtedly the sole occasion to date that I had entered an operating theatre without my usual swaggering confidence. Exuding self-assurance was the obstetrician's role here, but what really struck me was the air of calm that emanated from Sarah herself. Her pain had gone now and she could feel nothing below her breasts. Just as well, since they were painting her naked body with cold iodine solution from nipples to knees.

I watched as the sponge swirled over her breasts, around the smooth contours of her protuberant belly, then deep into the crevices of her groin. Soon light blue linen covered her chest, flanks and pubic hair before a sticky plastic sheet sealed the drapes against her body. The surgeon gave her a muted indication that the preparations were ending with 'We are going to get started now Steve is here.' Was that comment intended to camouflage the fact that they had waited too bloody long? Or was that just my paranoia? At this point I squeezed Sarah's hand, kissed her forehead, then fixed my gaze on the one and only operation that I ever found emotional. Empathy had arrived at last.

The liability insurance premiums for obstetrics are higher than for all other specialties, and it was always obvious to me why this was the case. Obstetricians are very direct in their approach, their knife slicing directly through skin, fat and abdominal muscle to the base of the dilated uterus, with little regard for bleeding. Late in pregnancy, blood volume is expanded, so, unlike my Jehovah's Witness adventure, a little bleeding is neither here nor there.

The blade kept on slicing within millimetres of my son's eyes and brain. After a skilfully judged, full-thickness incision through the uterine wall, in went the index and middle fingers of both hands to stretch the hole wide open. Digits are safer than cold steel around the baby's head. From knife to skin it took less than two minutes to deliver Mark's huge head. Although he looked very pissed off to be manhandled in this way, it should have been a relief to him not to have his head squeezed out through the claustrophobic pelvis by powerful contractions. As his torso emerged, the slimy umbilical cord spewed out from around the lad's neck and delivered itself.

All the while Sarah had been remarkably peaceful about the process. She squeezed my sweaty palm from time to time as if to reassure me, then, as the lad finally slithered from his nest, she said that it felt like a washing machine churning away in her belly. For a while our greasy blue bundle seemed lifeless. Newborn babies with airless lungs always appear slate grey, but I didn't recall that. All I remembered from our caesarean section just weeks earlier was that the slippery premature infant was almost dropped onto the floor as the umbilical cord was divided. Right now the placenta was the key to my anxiety. While still connected in the uterus, the baby doesn't need to breathe. Oxygen continues to be supplied to it, and blue blood returning to the heart is still diverted away from the unaerated lungs and back around the body. Blue had me worried, but it didn't trouble the special care team.

Once the umbilical cord was severed, Peter took our son to an incubator and sucked out his throat. Then we could hear him trying to breathe at last. There followed a howl as he inflated his lungs for the first time from their airless state. To me he still looked blue – I was clearly paranoid about blue babies – but Peter reminded me it was all to do with foetal haemoglobin molecules. A few more breaths and the colour improved. While the placenta was being scraped out and the uterus repaired, Peter handed Sarah her warm and now pink baby boy, and she burst into tears. Stupidly I needed to ask why she was crying and received an obviously feminine response – 'Because I'm so happy.' Twenty-six sleepless hours of painful labour were dispelled in an instant by the miracle of childbirth.

And what were her next words? 'Is your patient OK? Shouldn't you go and check?'

Sarah's wholly unselfish remark affected me deeply. This was the real reason St Thomas' had christened her Sister Beautiful – her beautiful selfless mind. So what on earth was she doing married to me, the Phineas Gage of cardiac surgery? That night I parked my demons and allowed myself some joy. The day had brought back empathy, something that usually caused me pain. The struggle to save poor Megan and preserve the dignity of her parents, then arriving in time to see my son born – it had all been an emotional rollercoaster. As Steinbeck wrote, 'It means very little to know that a million Chinese are starving unless you know one Chinese who is starving.'

I sat with Sarah for an hour in the recovery area, wrestling with my conscience about not having been there for Gemma's birth. I would spend a lifetime trying to make up for that. Then I thought about what Megan's parents must be going through, knowing that if she didn't survive it would be down to them. Whether it was through sympathy or compassion, I decided to relieve Neil Moat and spend some time talking with them on what must have been the worst day of their lives.

My baby was safe now. Theirs was lying under a cooling blanket now at 30°C, fighting for her life, with her brain's metabolic rate reduced by half to tide her over the profound anaemia. But I could see that we were winning. There was no bleeding, and her modest blood pressure was sufficient for the kidneys to produce urine – liquid gold, as we called it when the chips were down. Her grateful parents said God would reward me for this day's work. I said that he already had. I was blessed with a fine baby boy who had arrived at the end of Megan's operation. They interpreted this as divine intervention. Dr Gribben had already heard about the day's events and called into intensive care on his way home. Joy spread around the hospital that night, as my team were pleased for me too. Yet I was sad at the same time. And a bit lonely with my demons that night.

In the aftermath of Megan's miraculous recovery, the Jehovah's Witness Hospital Liaison Committee held a fund-raising campaign to acquire a cell saver machine for me. In turn I operated on their members from all over the country, combining the anti-bleeding agent aprotinin with the equipment they kindly donated. On one notable occasion a Jehovah's Witness with a leaking thoracic aortic aneurysm survived after being driven all the way from

Wales by his wife when he was refused surgery elsewhere.

Sarah and Mark came home three days after the birth, and I became even more sleep deprived than usual. Brian Gribben became Mark's godfather. The kindly neonatologist Peter Hope sadly died from cancer just a couple of years afterwards. Between us we had established a service for tiny premature babies in which I would open their chest and close a persistent ductus arteriosus – a common defect between the pulmonary artery and aorta – without taking them out from their incubator. This removed the risks of transfer from the maternity block to the main operating theatres, during which they lost heat. Mike Sinclair and I would travel to other regional premature baby units to provide the same service, but Mike eventually had to retire. A real character, he still has a great sense of humour and remains well.

Two years after her reoperation in Oxford, Megan's artificial mitral valve became infected. I was abroad when the family tried to contact me, and her closest cardiac centre was unwilling to attempt a third procedure without blood transfusion. She died from sepsis.

That cold winter's day in 1988 helped change my perspective on life and probably made me a better surgeon – not technically, needless to say, but as a result of becoming a much better human being. Love brings joy, yet until then I had been afraid to admit it.

7

danger

MANY INFECTIOUS DISEASES are transmissible through skin penetration, so wallowing in blood while handling sharp instruments is not without its dangers. Needle-stick injuries were a daily occurrence for me, but surprisingly enough, patients in most countries are not tested for blood-borne viruses before surgery. As a result, hospital staff are continuously exposed to risk through unsuspected contamination, a danger that is easily passed on to our families. On the flip side, irresponsible surgeons who are fully aware that they have hepatitis have infected hundreds of patients by failing to disclose the risk. Dangerous place, the operating theatre.

The No. 11 scalpel blade is sharply pointed. I used it at the end of every case to make those stab wounds through the body wall where the chest drains emerge. In the cardiac theatres in Oxford we had a polite and gentle Filipino staff nurse named Ayrin, who assisted me in my friend Steve Norton's case. As we finished an emergency case late one evening Ayrin was distracted by her runner nurse, who wanted to get the swab count done and make for home. She inadvertently thrust the blade end of the scalpel into my palm instead of the handle. As I reflexively grasped it, the glistening metal sliced through my rubber glove, breached my skin and painfully embedded itself in the muscle of my thumb. Bright red blood pissed out under the latex, forming a crablike pattern as it oozed through the tunnels of the rubber fingers. I squealed in shock and dropped the bloody implement, which fell to the floor like a dart and impaled itself bolt upright in the leather of my operating clog. After that I renamed her 'stab nurse Ayrin'.

Apart from my pain and the hilarity it provided for the rest of the team, this charade was no big deal. It was a clean blade, so I could not be contaminated with any blood-borne virus. Nothing was said nor done about the incident, except I was forced to leave the operating table and seek first aid. As I backed away, I thanked the mortified stab nurse for her help with the case. With time, a great deal of experience and progressively improving spoken English, 'stab nurse Ayrin' became sister in charge of the cardiac operating theatres.

For most operations I would work with two surgical assistants and a scrub nurse who slapped the instruments into my palm in an automated fashion that involved little forethought or deliberation. They knew all the steps of the operation as well as I did. I just presented my palm upwards and reflexively grasped whatever was thrust into it. My gaze was never diverted from the heart, unless to give an order. The surgeon conducts the whole team like an orchestra – 'Give the heparin, go on bypass, get the pressure down, come off bypass, give the protamine' – and the process benefits enormously from the finely honed skills of a consistent team.

We made every effort to look after each other, but the varied assortment of sharp instruments posed a constant threat. Used blades and needles are contaminated with the patient's blood, and we had little idea about the personal history of the vast majority. The stainless-steel needles are curved, usually presented on the end of a long metal needle holder and very sharp. They easily prick through thin rubber gloves, and at least twenty-five different blood-borne viruses are known to be transmissible. After operating for more than forty years covered with other people's fluids and enduring innumerable occasions when needles or blades drew blood, I generally regarded myself as immune to everything. Others were not as fortunate.

All operating theatre staff are immunised against hepatitis B, but some – like me – are non-converters who never develop the protective antibodies. In the early 1970s, when I worked in the famous Liver Unit at King's College Hospital, I was constantly exposed to hepatitis patients and their bodily fluids. Patients with cirrhosis of the liver develop varicose veins in their gullet called oesophageal varices. My brother David was a consultant in the Liver Unit and became a great expert at injecting these veins with sclerosing agents, and as a junior doctor I was called upon to stop the bleeding if they ruptured. When the patient started to vomit litres of hepatitis-contaminated blood, my job was to blindly pass a sausage-shaped balloon down their gullets as far as the stomach, the aim being to inflate it under pressure to compress the bleeding veins before they exsanguinated. Before too long the black digested blood poured out of their backsides and the nurses had to clean it up. Many terrified souls gave up the ghost and died at this point. Others absorbed the blood from their gut and turned bright yellow. More often than not, alcohol had been the problem.

For needle-stick injuries or blood in our eyes we would receive injections of hepatitis B immunoglobulin to counter the viral load, followed by a booster injection of hepatitis B vaccine. Despite repeated injections, this never seemed to impact on my own antibody levels. Moreover, there was no treatment for hepatitis C. We just had to wait and see whether we developed cirrhosis later in life. If the booze didn't get us first, that is.

I was tested for the hepatitis viruses every year to make sure I could not pass them on to my patients. But swimming in blood doesn't suit everyone. Needle-stick injuries petrified the nurses, and the extended periods of uncertainty caused them and their families hours of fear and anxiety. One German study showed that 80 per cent of the victims of needle-stick experienced high levels of stress about their future, damaging their personal relationships and screwing up their sex lives. Some even developed post-traumatic stress syndrome, which could only be helped by knowing whether the patient involved was a virus carrier or not. Yet testing without the patient's consent was not allowed. Many who were hepatitis positive through drug addiction or sexual promiscuity were not about to disclose their secrets. Sod the staff who were meant to care for them.

As the senior registrar at the Hammersmith Hospital in west London, I was always the one designated to operate on the intravenous drug abusers, not least because of my insight from King's. To be honest, I didn't even bother to ask permission to test their serology beforehand. I just assumed that they were all hepatitis positive, and told the nurses to expect it and take precautions. In the late 1970s this involved double-gloving and wearing impermeable hoods, gowns and goggles. 'Pigs in space' I used to call them, as they looked all set for a moonwalk. But at least they felt safer. I changed nothing, carried on as normal and generally was fine. Ironically the spacemen and women were at greater risk of needle-stick because their dread of exposure led to a nervy departure from protocol. I didn't even double-glove – it both failed to stop needle-penetration and reduced my tactile sense. It was like a paranoid student wearing two condoms then not enjoying sex, as in the days before my head injury took away fear. Life was much simpler after that.

Every time I operated on a drug addict with infected heart valves, my usually keen assistants seemed to fade into the woodwork. Some had a migraine, some had doctor's appointments. Others just said, 'No way – if you want to do it, just go ahead.' The consultant surgeons took the view that addicts were not worth the time spent in theatre as they always returned to injecting with reused needles and syringes in dirty public lavatories. With further foul abscesses at their injection sites, they would simply go on to infect their artificial valves within months of the operation. Sadly, this scepticism was justified, although it hardly seemed compassionate. Over the course of my whole career I only operated on one addict who did what he promised and gave up. But unlike my sanctimonious colleagues I didn't have a God complex. I had no wish to be judgemental.

Perhaps I lacked objectivity because I had a school friend whose miserable childhood was followed by a descent into the abyss of heroin addiction to escape from it all. The two of us used to go and watch Scunthorpe United, but he was soon dragged under by psychosis and received no help whatsoever – ten minutes with his GP and a prescription for Valium tablets didn't really cut it for schizophrenia. A couple of hours of heroin-induced euphoria was his way of coping, but eventually it killed him. The last time I saw him he was covered in abscesses and had septicaemia, kidney failure and a heart full of infected crap. They'd just let him go.

By the time I got these young people into an operating theatre they were always desperately sick, their blood boiling with the bacteria and viruses that could destroy any and sometimes all of their heart valves. Because the right side of the heart received the bacteria from their injected veins, it was often the tricuspid valve that disintegrated first. The infected valve leaflets would be covered in lumps of fibrin, resembling seaweed floating in and out of the right ventricle. We called these lumps 'vegetations' – they looked bad, often smelled like a sewer, and bits would break off to produce abscesses in their lungs.

I had already seen how surgeons in New York's borough of the Bronx handled this problem. The first time I told Professor Bentall at the Hammersmith that I was determined to take an addict to theatre against his advice, he asked which prosthetic valve I was going to use. He expected me to say a pig valve, but I surprised him. I said that I was just going to remove the crap and not bother to replace it, and that if the addict stayed clean for six months I'd take him back and put a pig valve in then. To my great surprise, the New York addicts normally coped without a tricuspid valve for several months, perhaps because it had not functioned as a valve for a considerable time beforehand. But the Americans hadn't yet published anything about their success in this arcane field because nobody was interested in drug addicts. As a result, Bentall thought I was crazy when I insisted that so-called valvulectomy was the way forward.

Certainly, most addicts survived tricuspid valvulectomy, but their cardiac output and exercise tolerance were limited. With free reflux of blood from the right ventricle back into the venous system, the liver would distend, swell and become painful. Should they decide to stop injecting, they eventually earned a brand new valve. If not, they faded away with right heart failure, abdominal pain and repeated episodes of sepsis. I did several tricuspid valvulectomies at the Hammersmith. All were cured of endocarditis, but none quit their heroin habit nor survived long enough to receive their pig valve. In that respect, I saved the NHS a couple of thousand pounds each time and eased my own conscience by taking them on in the first place. I never put the risks to myself before the needs of the patient, but I remained conscious of the fact that others were frightened for their own safety. The problem was, the more anxious they felt, the more likely they were to screw up.

Summer 1987. I had exhausted the whole year's budget for cardiac surgery in Oxford and found myself locked out of my own operating theatre by the management. At the same time, a front-line cardiac centre in Saudi Arabia had a sick heart surgeon and needed a locum. No financial problems there, and they were keen to have me. Unfortunately, my wife Sarah was six months pregnant and moving house. Tricky timing, but I soon found myself under the hot desert sun with a fascinating workload and a great international team.

Soon after I arrived in Saudi, a ten-year-old boy was admitted to the centre with sepsis. Philippe was the young son of a high-ranking official at one of the European embassies in Riyadh. The lad had been sent to public school in England but repeatedly suffered bruising after trivial injuries, then spontaneous bleeding into his joints. The first suspicion was leukaemia, and everyone was relieved when this was ruled out. The next suspected diagnosis was the autoimmune platelet problem known as idiopathic thrombocytopenic purpura. Sarah had that, which led to her spleen being removed when she was a student nurse in London. Her symptoms were the same as Philippe's.

When this diagnosis was dismissed, he was found to be clotting factor VIII deficient – a haemophiliac, whose plasma level was around 5 per cent of what it should have been. Now he was dependent upon regular factor VIII infusions, which he'd started in London. It was there that his doctors recognised a heart murmur, and he was shown to have a small ventricular septal defect. The paediatric cardiologists said that it would probably close itself in time, so surgery wasn't necessary. That was a relief for the parents because cardiac surgery in haemophiliacs is complicated, or at least it was thought to be back in those days. Without shedloads of factor VIII, they bleed and bleed.

So why was he in hospital this time? For weeks the boy had been losing weight and feeling generally unwell, and by now he was skin and bone, a pathetic sight given his swollen and deformed joints. Even with the air conditioning on at full blast, he would sweat profusely during the night. Then he had rigors, shivering uncontrollably as if he were having an epileptic fit. He also had pains in the chest, worse when he breathed in deeply – pleurisy brought on by dead wedges of lung, what we call pulmonary infarcts from infected emboli.

An esteemed American paediatric cardiologist made the diagnosis in five minutes. Philippe had tricuspid valve endocarditis, together with an infected ventricular septal defect directly beneath it. He was already receiving a powerful combination of antibiotics, but the fever didn't settle. Serial echocardiograms showed proliferating infected vegetations on the valve, which might grow through into the left ventricle then cause a stroke. I was asked to close the hole in the heart and either repair or replace the torrentially leaking valve. Repair was easier said than done, with aggressive bugs chewing through the leaflets. But he was a child, so just chopping out the valve as with the drug addicts was not an option. If the worst came to the worst, I would sew in a pig valve.

I already knew about contaminated blood products and the AIDS epidemic in haemophiliacs. Between 1981 and 1984, 50 per cent of haemophiliac patients in America were infected with contaminated blood and many died during the following decade. The same happened in Oxford, where the litigation involved was still active in 2018. AIDS could have explained the boy's emaciated state, but endocarditis would do that too. The responsible way forward would be to test him for HIV and hepatitis so that we could warn the staff. This required the express permission of his parents, but only Philippe's mother had been seen in the hospital. I was asked directly whether I'd be willing to operate on the boy if he was HIV positive. Without hesitation I responded that of course I would – the poor lad had suffered so much in his short life and would certainly die within days if no one was prepared to intervene. I would set aside the danger to myself. That's what surgeons do. Or did.

The boy's French mother took immediate offence at the mention of AIDS in regard to her son, insisting that this had never mentioned by medical staff before and claiming that no one they had met through the haemophilia clinic had ever contracted HIV during their treatment. Which clinic did the boy attend? She wouldn't say. Had he been tested for hepatitis? Yes, and he didn't have it. My American colleague sensed a standoff and an impending meltdown. The woman was already stressed enough at the prospect of her son's surgery, and her husband was nowhere to be seen. This was Saudi Arabia – strict laws, different culture, and AIDS was a dirty word.

I scheduled the urgent surgery and resolved to warn the staff of the potential risks. But my focus was on managing his risk of bleeding. I needed to organise the liaison between the anaesthetists, perfusionists, haematologists and the blood bank. Were there any guidelines for heart surgery in children with haemophilia? Not in 1987. So we had to work it all out from scratch. How much factor VIII concentrate did we need to transfuse to raise his levels from negligible to normal and eliminate the bleeding risk? That depended upon his weight. How much more should we infuse during cardiopulmonary bypass and then post-operatively to maintain his blood level? Between us, we worked out a dose regime and ordered the stuff on an urgent basis from the drug company in the UK. I couldn't take him to surgery without it, so I asked that it be dispatched overnight. We decided to monitor his factor VIII levels every six hours in the days following the oper-ation and try to keep them normal for at least a week afterwards. I would also give him my magic medicine aprotinin during and after the surgery to keep his platelets sticky.

I asked Julie, a vivacious, fun-loving Aussie who was bloody good at her job, to act as scrub nurse for the oper-ation, and I told her that we didn't think he was hepatitis or HIV positive. Having said that, I couldn't absolutely guarantee it, but the mother had reassured us of the fact. There was general and widespread hysteria about AIDS at the time as it seemed that no antiviral treatments had yet been developed and the mortality rate was high, and many felt that it was unreasonable to operate on HIV-positive patients because they were destined to die whatever we did. Efforts to defuse the backlash against the gay community gained little traction in Saudi Arabia. Even Julie was uncharacteristically reticent at the prospect, but she agreed to handle the instruments and keep me safe. I simply told the team that we should take the same precautions – hit and miss though they were – that we would use for a hepatitis case. Perhaps the mother's insistence that serology was off limits should have told us something.

I had a cunning surgical plan for the boy. I intended to clear the infected debris from the larger of the two tricuspid valve leaflets, then partially detach it to provide access to the hole between the two ventricles. I would close that with a Dacron patch, then enlarge and restore the anterior tricuspid valve leaflet with a patch of his own pericardium. Surgeons always need to have a strategy, but unpredictability was the exciting part about emergency surgery. I would keep it simple. If the valve fell to bits, I would simply replace it – easier surgery that didn't take much thought or judgement. I just needed to avoid stitching near the invisible electrical conduction system where it passes close to the ventricular septal leaflet. Destroy that, and the boy would need a pacemaker for life.

When I operated, I focused on the technicalities of the procedure and what I needed from the heart–lung machine – when to cool the body, when to rewarm, when to drop the flow, when to increase it. I would check the potassium level in the blood and whether there was urine flowing into the bag. I concentrated on the dangers to the patient, not the risks to myself, but it was not that easy for the assistants. Hepatitis was bad enough, but inoculation with serum from an AIDS patient terrified the life out of most healthcare workers.

Yet Julie was her usual cheerful self that morning, radiating charm and calm. All the nurses wore gloves and plastic face shields whether they were standing at the operating table or not, and the runners would not handle the swabs, picking them up with long metal forceps, then dumping them in a plastic bin. Julie double-gloved, with a niqab covering her head and goggles to keep blood out of her eyes.

Philippe was a sorry sight, lying there with his deformed joints, gaunt frame and skinny limbs covered in bruises. So much for factor VIII replacement. I told Julie and my surgical assistants to stand back as the saw spattered bone marrow onto the drapes and copious volumes of straw-coloured fluid were dispatched into the sucker bottles from around the heart and lungs. Without a functioning tricuspid valve, the right atrium was tensely distended, and dark blood pissed out as I placed the purse-string sutures that formed a seal around the bypass cannulas. To avoid Julie coming into contact with the needles, I carefully set the needle holders down on a magnetic mat by the bypass tubing. She could avoid handling the contaminated needles by shaking them from the jaws of the holder directly into the sharps bin.

At first sight the tricuspid valve looked like a bunch of grapes and had the sickly smell of digesting protein. With an addict I would have chopped the whole thing out, but for a child I needed to construct a silk purse out of that sow's ear of rotting tissue. I became more optimistic once most of the vegetations were scraped away and dumped into a bottle for the bacteriology department, and Julie's tense shoulders had dropped perceptibly by now. She was more relaxed, conscious that I was making every effort to keep her safe. The anterior tricuspid leaflet had a large hole eroded through its middle, so I simply enlarged it to give myself a view of the ventricular septal defect beneath. The hole was also obscured by infective crap that I disposed of down the high-pressure sucker. It was vital that none slipped through into the left ventricle then found its way into the boy's brain.

I closed the hole in the ventricular septum with a Dacron leaflet, then replaced most of the body of the anterior leaflet with preserved cow pericardium. No drama, and the heart separated easily from the bypass machine with lower pressure in the veins. Once the boy was given antibiotics targeting the infecting organism, he ought to be in the clear. We were on the home straight, so the tension in the room started to dissipate. I took the No. 11 blade to make the stab wounds for the chest drains, then carefully and deliberately placed the scalpel on the magnetic mat so that Julie could dispose of the blade.

With drains and two pacemaker wires in place, I set about closing the breast-bone. The stainless-steel wires are pulled into place on the end of a thick, sharp needle that is manually driven through the bone. I held the shaft of the needle tightly in the jaws of a heavy metal needle holder, which is usually handed to me directly by the scrub nurse. For this potentially infected case, we'd agreed that Julie would place the holder down on the magnetic mat and I would take it from there to avoid hand-to-hand exchange of the lethally sharp instrument.

This was all going smoothly until Julie's attention was drawn away to count the swabs before the edges of the sternum were pulled back together. I set the needle holder down with the last needle fixed in the jaws but pointing upwards. I was watching the heart, not Julie. I expected her to pick it up directly and toss it into the sharps bin. But she was facing her runner, not me.

As I said, 'Here's the needle, Julie,' she swivelled on her standing stool, lost balance and reflexively thrust her hand down onto the operating table to prevent herself falling. Her palm came down hard on the sharp point of the bone needle held fast by the jaws of the holder, the bone-marrow-contaminated spike being driven deep into her palm. She screamed, although I couldn't tell whether this was from the pain or simply the awful realisation that she had a deep needle-stick injury. Probably both.

Julie stepped backwards from the stool and stared at her wounded palm. Her glove had been torn when she drew her hand away from the spike and the wound was now briskly pumping blood. I barked at her to let it bleed, naively believing, as most of us did, that any contamination would be washed out. She stared at me, her piercing dark eyes clear through the goggles, and I registered the mix of fear and anger as she stood offering the bleeding hand to me. As her blood dripped onto the floor she mumbled, 'For God's sake, why did you leave it with the sharp end sticking upwards?' I had no answer.

I felt as sick about those disastrous few seconds as Julie did. She didn't know about the haemophilia–HIV link. Her immediate concern was the hepatitis risk, but we could do something about that. I stepped away from the table, discarded my blood-caked rubber gloves and said, 'Let me help.' There was an old-fashioned approach whereby we used to suck on a needle-puncture wound to draw out the evil humours. Totally worthless, I suspect, but she didn't try to stop me. It must have been a bizarre sight as we stood together, with me sucking her hand. I told my glum assistants to get on and close the chest, then escorted poor Julie to the coffee room.

I sat her down still quivering with the shock of it all, while I gathered my own thoughts. I knew that there were written guidelines for hepatitis post-exposure prophy-laxis, and I quickly found the operating theatre's protocol book, which read:

Unless already known, the infectious state of the
source should be determined. Unless known to be
negative for hepatitis B and C viruses, post-exposure
prophylaxis should be initiated within one hour of
the injury. Prescribe a booster dose of hepatitis B
vaccine together with hepatitis B immunoglobulin for
added protection. There is no vaccine for hepatitis C
so treatment consists of monitoring for
seroconversion.

In other words, you just wait and see if you get it. That's why Julie was so pissed off. She had gone through all this before back home in Australia after a needle-stick during a heart transplant when the donor was discovered quite by chance to be a hepatitis carrier.

I went back to theatre and asked the anaesthetist to draw some blood from the child for serology testing, but he told me that this couldn't be done in Saudi Arabia without the mother's permission. My blood pressure was already too high, but it immediately shot through the roof.

'Just take the fucking blood,' I yelled. 'I'll write the forms and take it to the lab myself.'

On the request form I wrote: 'Desperately sick haemophiliac child after cardiac surgery. Need to know what we are treating. HIV and hepatitis status please.' The boy was still on the operating table, so right now I was his guardian. I just needed to convince the lab that the tests were in the boy's interest, which they were. But my motives were dishonest. Philippe was doing fine. It was Julie I was

concerned about. Hepatitis was bad enough, but AIDS
was a death sentence in the 1980s. So I left Julie with her
bleeding hand under a tap and set off to find the
laboratories.

I was expecting a confrontation about permission to
test for HIV, but it never materialised. AIDS was rare in
Saudi Arabia and the assays were new, so I guess that they
were eager to try them out. It was not the virus itself that
the assays measured but the antibodies produced by the
patient in response to the infection. Then the obvious
question – how soon could they let me know if the patient
was HIV positive? They said they'd call in a couple of
hours, but if the boy did have AIDS what should I do? I
felt a deep responsibility for Julie, not to mention genuine
affection. Her cheerful disposition had made my life
much happier than it might have been in a difficult
environment. One expression I often heard from my
beloved elderly mother was, 'Put yourself in their shoes.
Try to understand what it's like to be them.' She would
apply that principle to the sick, the disabled, the mentally
ill and the poor. Or should I say poorer. 'They all have
feelings,' she used to say. Those few phrases defined
empathy.

By the time I returned to the operating theatres some
shit for brains had terrified Julie by warning her that
Philippe could be an HIV carrier. Her sore hand now
bandaged, she was pleading for someone to do something,
anything, to dampen down her fear. I rang a colleague to
ask whether there were any American infectious disease
doctors in the city who knew about AIDS and could help

us. Then I needed to talk with the boy's mother. While Julie was in meltdown about the risk of contracting AIDS, Philippe's mother was desperate for news from the operating theatre. I guess my face had that worried look as I approached, because she burst into tears as soon as she saw me. I held out my hand to her with the words, 'He's fine, it all went well.'

First things first. I described what I had done inside that rotting heart and said she could soon sit with the boy for an hour or so. I asked whether Philippe's father would be joining her and was told that he was 'somewhere in Europe'. Non-committal. I had to get to the point. Given the infected blood-products scandal in the US and Europe, had anyone ever tested her boy for HIV? I apologised for pushing her on this, but explained that a young nurse had been contaminated with Philippe's blood and desperately needed reassurance that there was no risk of AIDS or hepatitis. My question was carefully worded so as not to require a verbal response. I was as much a psychologist as a psychopath, and simply watching the expression on her face would give me the answer.

It was like throwing a switch, as she quickly diverted her gaze to the blank wall. Next question. 'Please tell me. Does Philippe have AIDS?'

Defensively reverting to her own language, she softly murmured, 'Oui.'

I took her sweaty hand and gently asked her why she hadn't told us.

'Because you wouldn't have operated on him if you had known, and I didn't want him to die.' With that, the poor woman fell onto the bed and started to weep uncontrollably. It was not a happy day.

We had to quickly find some sort of treatment for Julie, but I had no idea what that might be as quite frankly I knew nothing about HIV. I had never previously thought about it, yet I needed a firm grasp on the way forward before I faced her. By amazing coincidence, only a few weeks earlier the US had approved an antiviral therapy for AIDS known as AZT. For needle-stick injuries involving contact with an infected patient, the recommendation was to give AZT as soon as possible after exposure, certainly within seventy-two hours for there to be any hope of success. The treatment had to be continued for a month, and the side-effects included kidney failure, nausea, vomiting and diarrhoea. When I pressed the lab for Philippe's serology, they couldn't tell me whether it was positive or negative. It was their first attempt. I pressed harder, asking whether they could rule out it being positive, but they said they couldn't. I wondered whether dilution of his blood by the bypass machine or the drugs we had used like heparin or protamine could have made any difference.

I resolved to tell Julie that the test was negative but insist as much as I could that she should go through the AZT prophylaxis regime anyway. Better be safe than sorry. I was hedging my bets here. It was a fine balance between trying to minimise Julie's distress and knowing the full implications of the mother's confession that her son was an HIV carrier. With other symptoms masked by the endocarditis, he might well have full-blown AIDS, and

I needed to warn the intensive care unit about that now as a single room and spacesuits would certainly be required. As far as the nurses were concerned, this was worse than smallpox or bubonic plague.

We drew a blank on finding AZT, having called the medical director of the hospital, whose reply went along the lines of 'What's AZT?' His main concern was that other patients would not pay to come to the hospital if they learned that it was harbouring an AIDS case. Worse still, he now wanted everyone who'd been in contact with the boy to be tested for AIDS too, and the theatre obviously had to be cleaned and fumigated before it was used again. I could see this deep-cleaning regime extending all the way back to the airport, so I made the decision that we needed to dispatch poor Julie back to Sydney as quickly as possible. That would have to be as soon as tomorrow for AZT to be effective. She was unlikely to be able to afford an expensive ticket bought the day before travel, and as I felt strongly that the hospital should cover that cost I'd have to confront them about that. If they wanted to keep the AIDS story quiet, they should help Julie to leave the country sharpish, preferably in business class.

When I found her again in the nurses' changing room, Julie was gently sliding into the abyss. For a young woman in her twenties, this incident felt like a death sentence. In 1987 no one could put a figure on the risk of contracting full-blown AIDS from a needle-stick injury. What we did know was that it would be quite some time – months or years – before she would know whether she was safe or not. In the interim, everyone would treat her like a leper. The no-touch technique. No one would share her towel, let alone kiss or make love with her, and I felt responsible for all that. It had been my patient. It had been me who'd asked her to scrub for the case. Worst of all, I'd put that instrument down with the fucking needle pointing upwards. If only we could have wound the clock back.

I didn't want the poor girl to go back to her room and have no one to talk to. She needed a drink and so did I. The only place to find illicit alcohol was in the doctors' compound, so I resolved to smuggle Julie back to my apartment after dark. When I explained to her that she needed AZT but there was none in Saudi Arabia, she just curled up into a ball and said nothing. I knew the cardiac surgeons whom she worked with at St Vincent's Hospital in Sydney and I resolved to call them on the way to the airport. They would take care of her. We would organise her ticket, so all Julie needed to do was pack her bags. Would she ever return to Saudi Arabia with the prospect of HIV infection hanging over her like the Sword of Damocles? I doubted it. The poor kid came to work that morning full of life. One wobble on her stool and she faced a lifetime of uncertainty.

The newly published US recommendations advised serial HIV testing for six months after the initial four weeks of antiviral drugs. And 'counselling', whatever that meant. She would either be HIV positive or negative, and in the meantime the waiting to find out would dominate her every waking hour. With that, Julie, the bottle and I settled down for the night, and I did what I always did for my patients. I suggested that the risks were very low and that things would seem better in the morning. What's more, she was going home in a business-class seat. Scant consolation, I thought to myself, and if she was caught sharing my room we would both end up in jail – or worse.

I tried to keep in touch with Julie over the following years. The antiviral therapy in Sydney made her dreadfully sick for weeks on end, and her happy life and cheerful disposition were replaced by self-imposed isolation and depression. She never wanted to see the inside of an operating theatre again. She drank too much, avoided relationships and apparently had to resort to shoplifting when the money ran out. Although she never registered HIV positive, the trauma of that needle-stick and the fear of AIDS almost destroyed her. Almost, but not quite.

Ten years later I met her unexpectedly at a conference in Melbourne, where she was a heart failure nurse. She had seen my name on the programme posted in the hospital and was keen to let me know that she had a life again. It was an emotionally charged reunion because I had never forgiven myself for that innocent mistake with a viciously sharp needle. We found a fine bottle of blood red Australian merlot and she laughed a lot when I told her about the 'stab nurse' in Oxford. This was a far cry from the abominable Jeddah juice and that dreadful night with the bleeding hand.

Philippe died from AIDS just months after his operation. Of the many haemophiliacs exposed to HIV through blood products in the UK, 1,056 became HIV positive, 31 developed full-blown AIDS and 23 died. Had the blood-products industry and gay groups not refuted the evidence accumulated by the US Centers for Disease Control in 1982, much of this could have been prevented. I went on to insist that all our cardiac surgery patients in Oxford be tested for hepatitis and HIV as a matter of routine. This suggestion soon hit the buffers. Irrespective of the myriad of blood tests we did as a matter of routine, those for dangerous viruses could only be performed with the patient's explicit consent. Why? Because the potentially life-threatening diseases carried by some were associated with their personal habits, which – it was held – were no one else's business. My operating theatre staff seemingly possessed no rights.

I had no intention of being discriminatory or rejecting seropositive patients, but I wanted those in the front line like Julie to have the opportunity to protect themselves or indeed make their own choice as to whether they were willing to participate in the surgery. In my view, it was fair to test everyone whose blood we would pass between us, so I stuck to my guns. In my view, all patients benefited from their surgical team being protected, so if the system was not prepared to start routine testing I was not going to consent to annual hepatitis testing either. This precipitated a row with the medical director about hospital policy and fucking regulations. Anything but the welfare of my team.

From the safety of their desks, the General Medical Council declared that 'serology testing solely for the bene-

fit of the healthcare worker is unlawful.' Yet if our nurses
or perfusionists, who wallow in blood daily, inadvertently
contracted hepatitis or AIDS from an untested seropositive individual they could pass it on to others – their
spouse, their children or even other patients. It made no
sense whatever not to know what we were up against. So
I threatened a blanket ban on all categories of patient
who were deemed high risk for positive serology, claiming
that it was in the interest of the wider public. We all know
what that meant, but needless to say this was a hollow
threat. It was like a debate at the Oxford Union.
Meanwhile, panic about HIV was spreading. Those in
daily contact with blood, sharp instruments and complex
equipment simply had to be protected.

Over the years I went on to operate on a number of
HIV-positive patients without using spacesuits or
double-gloving. I felt it important for me to keep
everything as routine as possible, because it was those in
a state of nervous excitement who generally had the accidents. The World Health Organization estimated that
66,000 hepatitis B, 16,000 hepatitis C and 1,000 HIV
infections were caused in medical or nursing staff by
needle-stick injuries in the year 2000 alone. While 10 per
cent of hepatitis B-positive needle-sticks eventually
infected the recipient, the risk for hepatitis C was less than
2 per cent and for HIV it was just 0.3 per cent. But blood
from terminally ill AIDS patients was substantially more
infective. So Julie was lucky. Antiretroviral therapy and
prognosis for AIDS have improved greatly during the last
twenty-five years, yet the process of needle-stick prophy-

laxis remains onerous, uncertain and unpleasant for those involved. I eventually retired 'clean', despite hundreds of needle-sticks throughout my career. 'Stab nurse Ayrin' battles on as senior sister.

It was not until October 2018 that an official inquiry was opened into what the press deemed the worst-ever NHS treatment disaster. The proceedings began with testimonies from people who'd been infected with HIV and hepatitis. In a video played to the courtroom, one man described how he felt that he had lost his whole life after finding out at the age of forty-three that he'd been infected with hepatitis C as a child, when he was given an injection of infected blood products after a swollen knee was mistakenly diagnosed as haemophilia. One woman stated that she'd caught AIDS through her deceased husband, who was a haemophiliac. 'We were silenced and we kept quiet,' she said. As many as 30,000 patients who had received straightforward blood transfusions were also infected. Whole blood and blood products came from 100,000 paid donors in the United States, many of whom were prison inmates or from high-risk groups.

Why did this happen? Because the NHS was struggling to keep up with demand for treatment – a resources issue, as usual. As a result, around 5,000 patients with haemophilia and other bleeding disorders were infected over twenty years; half that number subsequently died. The UK government's legal team admitted that 'it was clear things happened that should not have happened.' Speaking on behalf of the Department of Health and Social Care in England, Eleanor Gray QC said, 'We are sorry. This happened when it should not have done.' Tell that to Philippe's mother, to Julie in Australia, or to me and the thousands of other NHS staff who remained at risk of contamination because the whole scandal was covered up.

8

pressure

FROM A SURGICAL PERSPECTIVE, small children with congenital defects in their tiny hearts are far more technically challenging to operate on than grown-ups, so our cerebral cortex and brain stem to fingertips axis has to be finely honed. Our empathy button also needs to be in the 'off' position – if only temporarily. We are all subject to transmitted anxiety, whereby someone else's fears are transmitted to our own mind. Body language, wobbly words and overt displays of emotion all figure in this process, no more so than when we talk to parents about operating on their child.

To maintain objectivity, the paediatric surgeon's psyche requires an invisible brick wall to deflect the misery, terror and panic vibes. This shouldn't be interpreted as callous or psychopathic, because it's not. Quite simply, the ability to resist the pressure of these emotions emanating from others is an acquired defence mechanism without which we couldn't do the job. Operating on other people's children is a peculiar responsibility.

According to new research from Cambridge University,

people acquire empathy through their upbringing and environment. What the Cambridge psychologists did was to analyse the genetics of 46,000 people who were asked to respond to a questionnaire designed to demonstrate empathy levels. They found that just 10 per cent of the variation between people's compassion and their ability to respond appropriately to the feelings of others was genetically based. Women are more empathetic than men. Given that empathy is an acquired trait, it broadly explains how doctors and soldiers learn to avoid it when they have to. I had a hugely empathetic mother, but when it came to children's hearts I learned to dispel the influence of her DNA. Clearly it is not a static phenomenon. When the pressure abates, empathy can return. And empathy at work is not the same as empathy at home. I was constantly concerned for my own children, particularly when my son Mark became a competitive rugby player, then drove as stupidly fast as I did.

As you might imagine, there was vastly more to establishing a children's heart surgery programme in Oxford than merely being able to perform the operations. My experience of congenital heart surgery with Kirklin and Pacifico, then a stint at Great Ormond Street Hospital in London, gave me the confidence to consider the prospect. Nothing gave me as much pleasure as watching sickly blue babies with terrified parents leave the hospital pink with happy families – mums, dads, grandparents, siblings all relieved of that crashing weight on their shoulders and never forgetting what their surgeon did for them. This was my motivation.

The commitment was huge in terms of time, energy and emotional commitment, but it gave me intense satisfaction. I had superbly dedicated children's cardiologists, anaesthetists and intensive care doctors behind me to relieve the pressure. Then, from a selfish standpoint, paediatric cardiac surgery lent Oxford an element of prestige that the rival Cambridge centre at Papworth lacked, something to offset their first-rate transplant programme.

Because we started from nothing, we remained the smallest paediatric cardiac centre in the UK, but goodwill and massive charitable donations built us the fine Oxford Children's Hospital. We had world-class obstetrics, neonatal intensive care and other paediatric surgical specialities alongside, everything we needed to provide the critical infrastructure for safe heart surgery.

Age eventually mellowed my perspective on professional life. I was recently preparing to give a talk in flooded Houston the week after the devastating 2017 hurricane and long after I had stopped operating on children. Sifting through my secretary Sue's print-out of the slides I found an envelope that she hadn't mentioned, one that had travelled with me all the way to the Texas Heart Institute. The letter within read:

Dear Dr Westaby,
I hope you are well! My name is Cara and you operated when I was 10. I must admit it is only in the last couple of years that I have started to understand how difficult and pioneering the Ross procedure was

and how lucky I am to have recovered the way I have.
I have recently completed my Batchelor of Psychology
degree. At my last appointment with my cardiologist,
he told me that I am healthy enough to have children
and am unlikely to need more surgery in the
foreseeable future. I understand that this result was
very improbable at the time of my first and second
operations and would like to thank you most
sincerely from the bottom of my heart for giving me
the opportunity to experience this life. I am visiting
the UK with my partner showing him the important
places from my childhood. As you and the John
Radcliffe are top of that list, I felt it important to
pop by.

    Lots of love,
    Cara xxxx

But I wasn't in the hospital at the time and so I never got
to meet grown-up Cara. Sue had taken the letter and
slipped it in with my papers for the trip. There was no
contact address, no way for me to tell Cara how much I
appreciated her message. Some time ago I wouldn't have
given it a second thought. Just another thank you letter,
another day, another complex reoperation in a child. I
didn't put myself in her position, nor feel concern for her
petrified parents who probably thought that this third
epic could be her last. Did I even meet them? Or did I fly
in the night before and do the plumbing in the morning?
An anonymous technical exercise was what I preferred in
those days. Others did the talking. Now things were

different and I was bitterly disappointed to miss her. I felt strangely protective about her prospects for motherhood and sincerely hoped that her own child wouldn't inherit the same problems that she had suffered.

Cara had been born with left ventricular outflow obstruction and an aortic valve that was far too small. As a result, her heart muscle was dangerously thick and it had to work far too hard to force blood around her tiny body. Mum soon noticed that something was wrong. Breast feeding was a problem, not a pleasure. It began enthusiastically enough, but disintegrated into breathlessness and wailing. Cara had 'failure to thrive', as the doctors put it. She was an emaciated, miserable baby, not plump and cheerful as she should have been.

When someone took the trouble to listen to her heaving chest there was an obvious murmur, a harsh sound behind the breast-bone as the powerful little ventricle squeezed blood through a pinhole. With just the stethoscope, her lady GP couldn't know what the diagnosis was, probably a small hole in the heart that shouldn't be there. Unfortunately, that was not the case. The hole should have been there, but much larger and with a three-cusp aortic valve in it. So skinny Cara was a hospital case rather than a baby you could pat on the head and patronise the mother by saying that it will all get better. It wouldn't. If left alone, this would soon have become a fatal problem.

Cara was referred as an emergency by my enormously talented paediatric cardiology colleague Neil Wilson. Using an echo probe, he'd made the diagnosis in five minutes – critical aortic stenosis and borderline hypoplastic left heart syndrome. Put simply, a tight valve with a left ventricle that was too small and grossly thickened. As a first option, Wilson wanted me to open up the stiff, thickened valve, what we call an aortic valvotomy. This should improve the heart failure symptoms and enable the left ventricle to grow.

So I took little Cara to the operating theatre the same day, where her diminutive, pale body looked lost on the table-top expanse of shiny black vinyl. We covered her with blue linen drapes so only the breast-bone remained visible through the adherent plastic sheet. Beneath, those skinny ribs heaved up and down in time with the ventilator. There was little fat between skin and breast-bone, even less than at birth. My blade sliced through the layers in one stroke and sharp scissors bisected the length of the breast-bone with little resistance, and no need for the saw. The electrocautery singed the oozing bone marrow, and in went the smallest metal retractor.

In babies, the fleshy yellow thymus gland covers much of the front of the pericardial sac. We removed it, cut through the glistening grey membrane, and there was the struggling heart. Cutting into the pericardium of a baby is like opening a surprise birthday present. We can anticipate what we're going to find from the echocardiogram but it doesn't spoil the moment, much like entering the Woodstock Gate into Blenheim Palace near my home. I've done it so often, but each time the impact is breathtaking. Every baby's heart is different and unique in some way, never a disappointment but often intimidating; such were Cara's diminutive aorta and left ventricle, as underdeveloped as the echo had suggested. The aorta would only accept the smallest perfusion cannula for the bypass circuit, and we knew that the narrowed valve had fused cusps with a pinhole orifice, which we needed to make bigger. Her ongoing survival depended upon that.

Nothing is simple in neonatal heart surgery. There is substantially more fluid in the cardiopulmonary bypass circuit than in the baby itself, which poses some difficult questions. How much will it dilute the blood? How much flow does the baby need and at what temperature? And how much cardioplegia is required to stop a thick, walnut-sized heart?

A surgeon doesn't work in isolation, but I couldn't concentrate on the technical details if I was constantly having to tell my assistants what to do. Happiness is a consistent surgical team. Same people every case, the American way. People you can trust to do a good job, not a different face every time depending upon who is available. My enthusiastic international fellows were the answer, professionals who were eager to be there for every case because they wanted to learn. I was surrounded by top guys from the US, Australia, Japan and South Africa, although it didn't matter where they came from as long as they were keen. I certainly didn't need whinging registrars simply rostered to be in my theatre when they would have rather been off duty, all set to clock off when their European working time hours expired. Stocking up on rest does not make for a great surgeon.

With a clamp separating the perfusion cannula from the tiny root of the narrow aorta I made a transverse incision, carefully avoiding the orifices of the two main coronary arteries that emerge above the valve itself. Damage a main coronary artery in a small baby and it's curtains – no coronary blood flow, no muscle contraction, no circulation. There's absolutely no margin whatsoever for error. A normal infant aortic valve has three virtually transparent cusps. Those with congenital aortic stenosis often have two thickened and fused cusps. Cara had one rigid cusp – a rare volcano-like valve with an orifice so small I was surprised she survived birth as the thick left ventricular muscle could have easily fibrillated during the metabolic mayhem of delivery.

Now I needed to cut into it so that it would open as widely as possible. This required precise evaluation. Should I try to create three cusps like a normal aortic valve, or two cusps so that it would open like a bird's beak? The thickened collagenous lump was so deformed that I decided to go for the latter. Two carefully judged cuts from the pinhole out to the perimeter of the valve ring and it was done. Now it opened like a puffin's bill, but it was still thick and stiff. Although I knew we would be back to work on it again in time, this first step would provide better body blood flow and help the left ventricle to grow.

When I removed the cross clamp the heart began to wriggle and squirm in ventricular fibrillation. Then quite spontaneously it stopped and sat motionless in its fibrous cocoon. No problem – the bypass machine kept pumping warm blood around Cara's little body and I knew it would start again. A poke to the empty right ventricle with the tip of my forceps and it contracted just once in response, as if to say piss off, I'm enjoying the rest. Keen to move on to the next scheduled case, I prodded it again and asked for the pacing wires. The heart got the message. It didn't want the electrical shocks; it would rather get on and beat for itself. Blips on the monitor's arterial trace showed that it was ejecting some blood, but the heart was still empty at that point. I told the perfusionist to leave some blood in, and the arterial trace got stronger. The heart looked happier with the blockage relieved, so we weaned Cara from the circuit.

As it so happened, Cara's aortic valvotomy was the easy case for that day. The next baby was just two days old, with an aorta that literally stopped after the branches to his head and right arm – an interrupted aorta, as we call it – and a large ventricular septal defect between the two pumping chambers. After birth, babies with this condition can only survive as long as the ductus arteriosus, nature's temporary connection between the main artery to the lungs and the disconnected distal aorta, remains open. As a result, the upper half of the body may be pink with well-oxygenated blood while the lower half looks blue with deoxygenated blood from the pulmonary artery. A harlequin baby.

If the ductus arteriosus closes soon after birth – as it is programmed to do – the whole lower half of the body is starved of blood flow and the baby dies. Only an infusion of hormones to fool the ductus that the baby is still in the uterus can keep it alive. My job was to dissect out and join up the tiny ascending and descending parts of the aorta, making sure that all the self-closing ductus arteriosus tissue was removed. These tubes are around the size of a child's drinking straw, so the process is more easily described than done. It can only be achieved with the baby cooled down to 18°C and the circulation stopped altogether.

The cooling took around thirty minutes on the bypass machine, so I set about closing the hole in the heart with a patch of Dacron fabric, like sewing a button on a shirt but working inside a thimble. There is always a significant gap to span between the two ends of an interrupted aorta. The distal end begins way down in the back of the chest and has multiple branches to the chest wall. Consequently, it must be mobilised carefully and pulled forward. At the same time, it is important not to cut too many branches, as this can compromise the blood supply to the spinal cord.

Lots of technical considerations make this a complicated procedure, during which there is no blood flow to the brain or heart muscle. It's a race against the clock. Once I had created the new aorta, we started up the heart–lung machine again and rewarmed the infant back to 37°C. It was then that the problems started. Blood began to well up from the dark recesses of the chest. Not torrential, but persistent.

Rewarming would normally take around another thirty minutes, giving me the chance to go out and relieve my aging bladder after I'd invited my assistant to stand in for me. But not this time. I needed to find the troublesome bleeding and stop it, not easy when it comes from way back against the vertebral column. Eventually I found the bleeding artery on the chest wall where a tiny titanium clip had fallen off. By then we had stopped and restarted the bypass machine on several occasions because we had difficulty in retracting the heart out of the way. Now it was objecting strongly, beating but not pumping. When three separate attempts to separate from bypass ended in failure, I thought the baby would not survive.

In those days as many as one in five of these babies would not get through surgery. So should I just give up and go home? It was now six in the evening, when everyone else was finishing work. The end of the day for me meant the end of the baby's life – and the end of the world for the poor parents. So we battled on. Supportive drugs and more time on the machine did not make this heart any stronger, and a fifth of the left ventricular circumference now consisted of a Dacron patch, which, needless to say, didn't contract. All of this, together with repeated muscle stunning through periods without blood flow, meant that the odds were stacked against us. Without mechanical circulatory support, death was inevitable.

There was only one circulatory support device suitable for small children. This was the Berlin Heart, an external air-driven pumping system that I had once used to keep a boy with a heart muscle disease alive until we transplanted him in Oxford. I had paid for that apparatus and the Lear jet from Germany from my own research funds. But the

NHS would not pick up the tab for this equipment, so I didn't have a device for the baby dying on my operating table.

What I did have was an adult circulatory support system that had been sent from the US for us to test. This Levitronix centrifugal pump was the last of five donated free of charge, and every one of the others had saved a patient in shock who would otherwise have died. Could I adapt this adult system for a newborn baby? It had certainly never been done before, we didn't have regulatory approval to use it in children and there were several worrying technical issues to overcome.

As with the heart–lung machine, the Levitronix circuit contained more volume of fluid than a child's whole circulation, so we would have to fill the tubing with blood to avoid excessive dilution. Next, this pump normally provided between five to seven litres of blood flow per minute, more than enough for a 70 kg man but far too much for a 1.7 kg baby. We'd need to switch the flow rate way down and compensate by increasing the level of anticoagulation to prevent clot formation. The flip side was that this would increase the risk of bleeding into the chest or brain. Finally, the nurses in paediatric intensive care had no experience of the device, so an adult team would have to be called in to help.

Every time I did something unconventional like this, someone complained to the management and I was threatened with the sack. Did that ever impact on my thought processes? No. We have an NHS that publishes surgeons' death rates but fails to provide the equipment necessary for rescuing lives. Where is the morality in that? My perfusion team were up for the challenge, as no one wants to see a waxen dead newborn washed clean and placed in a shroud at the end of a long operation, least of all the nurses who have to deal with the body long after the bean counters have gone to the pub to celebrate their cost savings.

To connect the Levitronix circuit I simply left the small aortic perfusion cannula in place but switched the venous drainage pipe from right to left atrium. After trying one last time to separate from bypass but failing miserably, we stopped the heart–lung machine and I swiftly made the adjustments. At this point, the baby hovered between life and death for one minute, two minutes, then three minutes. Any more time spent at normal body temperature without circulation and his brain would have suffered irreversible damage.

The circulatory support system was connected in less than four minutes and the spinning rotor switched on to provide one litre of blood flow per minute. We still had a live baby, albeit one with low blood pressure and lacking a pulse. Unlike the pulsatile Berlin Heart, the Levitronix pump provides continuous blood flow. Managing pulse-less people in the intensive care unit is fraught with diffi-culties, but my adult circulatory support nurses were on their way back to the hospital. As we closed the tiny chest over the pipes, I had no real expectation that we could win this one. Many things could still go wrong, yet in my mind any chance of recovery was worth the effort. The alternative was an interminably miserable interview with bereaved parents in the dingy relatives' room, trying to convey something I didn't fully understand myself. I had been there before, often on behalf of less robust bosses who couldn't face the prospect themselves.

I sat with the nurses beside the cot, watching the sun go down, then long into the night. None of those alongside me were 'on duty'. We were simply doing our best for this family and taking the usual crap for it. 'Should you really be using this pump in a baby?' I'd be asked. Answer: 'Would you prefer for the child to be in the mortuary? If so, you're in the wrong job.' My brain followed on with, 'So go shit yourself,' but I wouldn't verbalise that. Cara was in the cot next door, with her anxious parents each holding a tiny hand. She was still sleeping in drug-induced La La Land, but was doing fine.

It took three days of circulatory support with the Levitronix system for the boy's tiny heart to recover. As soon as we were convinced it was strong enough, we took him back to the operating theatre and removed all the intimidating machinery. Two weeks later he left hospital with happy parents. Had we not had that last freebie from the company in the States, there would have been a funeral not a happy homecoming. It was charity-shop healthcare.

I remember the day that Cara left hospital for one curious reason – I repaired atrial septal defects in the hearts of three siblings that day. Why? Because their mother was so distraught at the prospect of her kids being operated on that she couldn't decide who should go first or last. To limit her suffering, the children's intensive care unit agreed to take all three on the same day and brought in extra nurses to assist.

It was four years before I saw Cara again. During that time Dr Wilson kept her under close surveillance, with echocardiography every six months. At first she made great progress. The heart failure disappeared, her feeding improved immeasurably, and she blossomed and grew into an active toddler. Her left ventricle grew too. Then gradually things started to slow down again. The murmur directly behind the breast-bone grew louder once more, with the echo pictures showing the aortic valve to be stiff and narrow as the muscle became thicker. There were long faces in the clinic, and it was time for another proce-dure. Wilson decided against the less invasive balloon dilatation, so I took her back to the operating theatre to do the best I could before she started school.

When I exposed the valve it had grown to some extent, but the orifice was tight again. As before, I cut outward from the restricted hole with a sharp scalpel blade to mobilise the two thickened cusps. Under the valve itself the muscle was thick and obstructive, so I cut away a channel to enlarge the outflow from the ventricle. It looked better but didn't give me much cause for optimism, and I remember thinking that it would only last a couple more years. Cara bounced back and skipped happily out of the hospital, although her parents knew she would have to return. She had been born with a self-destruct mechanism and next time there would be no alternative but to replace the valve.

There are no artificial heart valves small enough to use in young children, but there is one valve replacement operation that can be done, a complex, intimidating procedure that few surgeons ever attempt. I learned it from its originator, my old boss Donald Ross at the National Heart Hospital. Ross came up with the ingenious idea of removing the patient's pulmonary valve and transposing it to the aortic position, then replacing the pulmonary valve on the low-pressure side of the heart with a pulmonary valve taken from a dead donor. The procedure worked well in adults, but even Ross had never attempted it in a small child.

After learning the steps and pitfalls from Ross, in 1995 I was the first surgeon to perform the procedure in a baby. This boy was found to have a heart murmur following an emergency caesarean section. Within hours the struggling left ventricle had failed and he was turning blue with low blood flow, so I rushed him to theatre to do exactly what I had done for Cara – put him on a heart–lung machine, then cut into the valve to relieve the obstruction. Just like Cara, he was one day old. The echo pictures the following day showed an improvement in flow, and after several days in intensive care the family were allowed home.

Six weeks later the valve seemed tighter than ever and the left ventricle contracted poorly. The boy was going to die if nothing could be done. Faced with that prospect, I decided to take the bull by the horns and risk Mr Ross's operation, although he would probably have thought me bloody mad to attempt it in such a tiny heart. Then there was the added issue of sourcing the spare part, an infant pulmonary valve from the autopsy room.

We didn't know whether the switched valve would grow in its new position, yet we were certain that the dead donor pulmonary valve wouldn't. So I needed to oversize it, but we were never going to be offered a row of dead babies to choose from. We were lucky to obtain the valve from a three-year-old accident victim – misery for its poor parents, although the knowledge that their lost child had saved another baby's life provided a small crumb of comfort. The valve would wear out one day, but at least it would take the boy through to his teenage years.

It was an intensely worrying case right from the start. The left ventricle was so poor that the stiff little lungs were floating in a pool of straw-coloured fluid. There was more heart failure fluid within the pericardial sac, which spurted out as soon as I made a hole in it. Then the aorta was so narrow that the smallest perfusion cannula almost blocked it. My first attempt to insert it missed the tiny incision altogether and we were sprayed with blood. It went in on the second attempt, then I put the baby on bypass and stopped the heart with cold cardioplegia solution. What followed was just about the most nerve-wracking heart operation in the book, miniaturised and without precedent. But it was still the Ross procedure, not mine.

I cut across the aorta below the perfusion cannula and proceeded to mobilise the vital coronary artery buttons, which were no larger than pinheads. These had to be re-implanted into the baby's own floppy pulmonary autograft without kinking or tension. Life depended on that.

There was no music in theatre and no one spoke unnecessarily. Every so often my anaesthetic colleague Mike Sinclair would put his head over the drapes and ask how it was going. 'Slowly. It's bloody difficult,' was my automatic response. Yet we were desperately working against the clock. The longer the cardiopulmonary bypass time and the longer the period without blood flow to the heart muscle, the greater the risk of death.

The step that made my adrenaline levels surge was the dissection of the pulmonary valve root out from the ventricular septum in proximity to one of the main branches of the left coronary artery. This required sharp dissection with a glistening scalpel blade less than a millimetre from a vital vessel buried in muscle – a bit like hanging a picture while trying to avoid a high-voltage electric cable hidden under the plaster. I knew where it should be but couldn't be certain. I almost lost my first adult Ross patient – a young mother of two small children – by occluding that invisible coronary artery with a stitch. Had she died, when instead she could have had a straightforward valve replacement at low risk, I would never have attempted another Ross operation.

After the agony comes ecstasy, at least it did in this case. I enlarged the outflow tract of the left ventricle and switched the valves, finally re-implanting the origins of the tiny coronary arteries back into the new aortic root. The donor valve then filled the gap created by removing the pulmonary root. Magic. We had succeeded within a reasonable time frame. What's more, the new valves didn't leak. Although I was a surgeon, when we took off the clamp to let blood back into the heart I felt more like a painter who had just put the finishing touches to his masterpiece. This remodelling of the whole outflow of the heart was a voyage of discovery. Ross had anticipated that the patient's own pulmonary valve would remain alive in the blood stream, giving it the potential for growth in children. Now we would find out. Could this at last be the solution for lethal aortic stenosis in babies?

The Ross procedure was the only operation I was consistently apprehensive about performing – and it's not difficult to understand why. Indeed many other surgeons found it far too intimidating in comparison with straightforward, low-risk aortic valve replacement for adult patients using a commercially produced valve off the shelf. Others who had a go sometimes made errors that proved fatal. But for small children, the only other option was to use an aortic valve from a dead donor, and this doesn't grow as they got older because it imbibes calcium and soon turns into a tube of chalk. On the few occasions when I backed away from the Ross operation and used an aortic homograft in a child, I usually regretted it.

Cara came back at the age of ten. She couldn't run or play with the other kids at school – simply walking across the playground made her breathless, giving her panic attacks as she felt she was being strangled. Then there was the crushing pain in the centre of her chest when she became excited about anything. Life was increasingly miserable for her, while her parents were consumed by the anxiety that inevitably comes with third-time heart surgery. Complex reoperations were always fraught with uncertainty and the prospect that we might terminate a young life, although in reality that rarely happened. Yet as I grew older and less able to assemble a consistent operating team, I became more conscious of the risks.

We discussed every case at a multidisciplinary team meeting before executive decisions were made. By then, Neil Wilson had become the country's leading light on balloon dilatation of narrowed valves in children. He would insert a balloon-tipped catheter into a leg artery and retrogradely feed it up the aorta under X-ray guidance. The latex balloon was then inflated under high pressure to split open the obstructive valve leaflets. Hopefully this would take place along the lines of fused valve cusps, but it didn't always work out that way. Sometimes the valve tore in the wrong direction, then leaked badly. Yet Wilson was so talented and bold with his catheters that he began to dilate valves like Cara's when the baby was still in the womb. Really scary stuff.

I was expecting the meeting, dominated as it was by cardiologists, to recommend an attempted balloon valvotomy for Cara – but it didn't. The technology of magnetic resonance imaging had recently been introduced, and the pictures they gave of her thickened, gnarled and rigid valve were detailed and depressing. There was no point submitting her to another general anaesthetic on a 'have a go' basis. I had already published an account of the first infant Ross procedure in the journal *Heart* and that's what the meeting wanted for Cara, not more temporising efforts.

Was there any alternative? Although Cara was small for her age, it might be possible to remove the valve, further enlarge the channel out of the ventricle and implant the smallest mechanical heart valve, possibly a much more straightforward operation – if third-time operations can ever be described as straightforward. But she'd have to take the anticoagulant drug warfarin for the rest of her life and would require a larger valve in a few years' time. Moreover pregnancy, although possible, would be a nightmare for her in these circumstances.

After the group discussion about which operation to do, Wilson came right out with it: 'A mechanical valve will leave her with the lifelong risk of stroke and anticoagulant-related bleeding. That's the coward's way out. You described the Ross operation in children. Just get on and do it.'

So that is what we did – and fortunately it went well. Our homograft bank found an adult-sized donor pulmonary valve that I hoped would last Cara indefinitely. When we followed the Ross operation in children over the years, we found that their own pulmonary valve did indeed grow normally in its new position. As a result we had some miraculous long-term successes. What's more, the donor valves lasted much longer than we expected in the right side of the heart because the pressure and stresses are much lower.

So finally, as I have no way of tracing her, here's my reply to the letter from Cara that I discovered in my papers at the Texas Heart Institute.

Dear Cara,

I was desperately sorry to have missed you when you came back to the hospital in Oxford. You must feel that you never met me during the rollercoaster of those three operations but please understand that I knew you very well. I wanted to let you know that I cared about you and your parents during those difficult times. You helped to prove how successful that Ross procedure could be. Donald is no longer with us but he would have loved to have heard your story. I wish you many successful pregnancies and a happy life. I hope someone sees this letter and tells you about it.

Love to you and the family,
Prof.

9

hope

GRIM REAPER TIRELESSLY STALKED the hospital corridors with his scythe, hoping for me to screw up. Sometimes I did, mostly I didn't, but I never let anyone go without a fight. My motto was Winston Churchill's message to the country in the dark days of the Second World War: 'We shall never surrender.' Winston's grave was the halfway point of my Blenheim Estate jogging – perhaps 'staggering' – circuit, which I'm too old for now. I would sit and talk with him on the bench donated by the Polish resistance. And there were always flowers there all year round, often with the message 'Hope springs eternal'. I had hope, my patients had it too, as did their loved ones. In the hospital, love, hope and triumph are bedfellows, while disappointment and grief lurk menacingly in the wings – or under my operating table. The difference between these extremes was skill, resilience and unstinting effort. Does that glorious trio still exist these days?

On a cold, miserable February morning I was about to take a patient off the bypass machine after an aortic valve replacement when a nervous blonde head poked through the operating theatre door. This time it was the paediatric cardiology registrar. Would I come straight away to the children's intensive care unit? There was a dire crisis. My patient's heart was beating vigorously, so my assistant came around to take over. With a sense of déjà-vu I backed away and peeled off my blood-caked gloves.

'It had better be an emergency' was the only thing I could say.

My registrar was a safe pair of hands, but through bitter experience I had learned that it was not a sensible time for me to leave. The intensive care unit was just a hundred yards down a straight corridor, past the accident department. The messenger moved quickly at a trot, betraying her considerable stress. By the time I arrived she was already holding the heavy door open, while the nursing sister held open a second swing door between the relatives' waiting room and the inner sanctum. It was a clear statement. We want you in here quick. And what kept you?

Green drapes were drawn around the bed, but through a parting I saw the frenetic activity and the fact that the stark tableau within spelled death. Someone announced, 'He's here,' but no one looked up. They were in the process of trying to resuscitate Sophie, a thin, deathly pale fifteen-year-old. Anaesthetists, cardiologists and paediatricians – all were huddled around the one body. My eye was drawn to the long wide-bore needle poking into her chest directly over the heart. A large syringe was withdrawing heavily blood-stained fluid, then pushing it out into a plastic bag through a three-way tap. So far there was half a litre of the stuff, which had been compressing the ventricles. The anaesthetist was rhythmically squeezing a black rubber gas bag, blowing in oxygen through corrugated plastic piping down into the girl's stiff lungs through the tube sticking out of her throat. I glanced instinctively at the monitor screen. Her heart rate was 130 beats per minute, much too fast; her blood pressure was half what it should have been, but that was OK – better low than nothing. Mercifully the girl was already deeply unconscious, completely unaware of being transfixed through the chest by that needle. Grim Reaper was trying to take her, but the resuscitation team wouldn't let go.

It was the start of the real battle, although she'd already been through multiple skirmishes. Her brown case-notes folder lay open on the table. The opening entry was from the district general hospital to which she had been first taken. It read:

Sunday 16 February. 11 pm. Fever, neck stiffness, headache and muscle pains. Started having knee and elbow pain on Saturday afternoon. Went to sleep it off but still present. Went to Dad's on Saturday evening when the temperature reached 104°F. Worsening headache, vomiting and generalised body ache. Stayed in bed yesterday. Today worsening headache despite 200 mg Ibuprofen x 4. Vomited three times. Now has neck stiffness and generalised limb pains. Heart rate 104. Blood pressure 95/50. Diagnosis viral illness but exclude meningitis. Pupils OK.

As if all this were not miserable enough, she then had to endure three unsuccessful attempts at a lumbar puncture by junior doctors, the aim being to tap a specimen of cerebrospinal fluid from the spinal canal, the same fluid that surrounds the brain. In meningitis, this crystal-clear fluid becomes cloudy with white blood cells and in the worst cases it looks milky, full of bacteria. I did lots of lumbar punctures as a houseman at Charing Cross, shoving the long needle in one direction then another, trying to find a way through into a narrow space past arthritic vertebral bones. The patients hated it and I hated it, but I always found the fluid in the end. Often lives depended on it. But Sophie's doctors had failed and given up, which was inexcusable. If it had been meningitis she would be dead already. Instead, they put in a drip in her arm to give her fluids and took blood for culture to see if there were any bacteria in her blood stream.

Over the next twelve hours Sophie became desperately ill. Antibiotics were given into the drip, but without isolating a bug it was all guesswork and her condition worsened. The next evening her blood pressure started to fall and her heart rate climbed to 120. Next, they transferred her to the coronary care unit of the district hospital, then by ambulance to our children's intensive care unit in Oxford. Powerful vasopressor drugs were needed to keep her blood pressure above 60 mm Hg as she deteriorated into septic shock. The next morning, the bacteriology laboratory reported a heavy growth of *Staphylococcus aureus* bacteria in Sophie's blood, a common organism that thrives on skin but is extremely dangerous when it enters the blood stream.

It was then that a painful hot red swelling appeared on the back of her right hand, diagnosed as septic arthritis by the intensive care doctors. An urgent cardiac echo was performed that evening by one of the unit registrars but was deemed unremarkable. Worryingly, this particular staphylococcus organism was found to be resistant to treatment with penicillin, so the antibiotics regime was changed. Sophie was becoming short of breath and began hallucinating. An urgent chest X-ray showed fluffy shadowing and fluid accumulating in both chest cavities around the lungs.

The following morning the plastic surgeons decided to drain the pus from the infected hand, believing it to be the source of the blood-stream infection. Or was the blood-stream infection the cause of the septic arthritis? Impossible to say, given that single snapshot in time and an 'amateur night' echo that had missed the point. Because she was desperately sick, the surgery was carried out with only local anaesthetic, which made it miserable – to say the least – for poor Sophie. But sure enough, the fluid evacuated from the joint did grow the same staphylococcus bug. Then another cardiac echo performed by Dr Archer showed fluid accumulating around the heart. She was becoming anaemic and needed more intravenous fluids to keep her blood pressure up, added to which her temperature chart was still swinging up and down like Wall Street on a nervy day.

One week after Sophie first came to Oxford, Dr Archer detected a new heart murmur. The echocardiogram showed the mitral valve to be leaking and yet more fluid around the heart. With increasing echo density, this fluid was beginning to look like pus, and she was now so anaemic that she needed a blood transfusion. Her anxious little family gathered around the bedside. Despite heavy-duty antibiotics, Sophie remained critically ill. Her mum Fiona and sister Lucy already believed that they would lose her, so they had moved into a room in the hospital. There followed more antibiotics, more fluids and more blood pressure drugs – but still no improvement. With the relentless swinging temperature, she suffered worsening delirium and terrifying nocturnal hallucinations. How sick can one kid get without an obvious diagnosis?

Next morning came the catastrophic deterioration that caused me to be summoned to her bedside. Sophie finally suffered terminal cardiovascular collapse and respiratory arrest, prompting a call for the paediatric resuscitation team and finally the heart surgeon. Without aggressive resuscitation measures she was dead at this point. First they had to intubate her windpipe and take control of her breathing, then relieve the pressure on her heart by drawing out the infected fluid that was compressing it, hence the big hollow needle and syringe. As her blood pressure started to improve, Archer took the echo probe to show me the cause of the crash. Sophie's mitral valve had been infected all along and had suddenly disintegrated under pressure. Huge lumps of infected proteinaceous material were dangling from it, ready to break free and fly off into her brain. Had she needed cardiac compressions, the likelihood was that these would have already detached and caused a massive stroke.

But now it was essential for her to go directly to the operating theatre to replace that buggered valve. No ifs, no buts, no debate. The honeymoon period with improved blood pressure wouldn't last. The infection was winning. Every time the left ventricle contracted – a frenetic 130 times per minute – more blood was refluxing backwards into the left atrium than passing forwards to the aorta. Sophie's heart was barely pumping any blood onwards and her lungs were filling with fluid. Either the previous echoes had missed this morass of teaming bacteria eating their way through the tissues or the bug was so damned aggressive that we were unlikely to succeed whatever we did.

The second planned patient of the day had been given premedication and was already on her way round to the anaesthetic room. The poor woman had to be turned back at the operating theatre doors, a dire experience for any anxious patient and their waiting family, all now psychologically prepared for heart surgery. I went back to the theatres myself and told them to get ready for an urgent mitral valve replacement in a desperately sick teenager. What was the name of the patient? I didn't even know that. I hadn't asked. Nor had I spoken with the frantic parents and sister. There simply hadn't been time.

Having announced the change in plan, I returned to the intensive care unit. Archer was in the relatives' room with them all, a highly intelligent family who had been told that Sophie was dying. He had already done the difficult bit and explained the bad news, and profound worry was now etched on three desolate faces. How do you make the impending death of a child any easier? Give them some hope, maybe. That magic word. Hope was my job, and with my ingrained optimism and lack of self-doubt I explained that although an infection had completely destroyed the mitral valve, we could replace it. We were fortunate to have the chance of getting into an operating theatre quickly and needed to do so as soon as possible. There was one last thing to warn them about – if Sophie was given an artificial valve she would have to be anticoagulated with warfarin for the rest of her life. Warfarin is needed for prosthetic valves to reduce the production of clotting proteins by the liver. I sidestepped further questions by saying I was going to push Sophie around to the theatres myself as we couldn't wait for porters. It had to be now.

We bypassed the anaesthetic room and deposited Sophie's unconscious body directly on the operating table. Most of the necessary cannulas and electrodes were already in place to hook up to the operating theatre monitors, my instruments were all laid out on blue linen – a paediatric set and an adult set, because she was in between – and the nurses were ready. The white fluffy swabs were carefully counted and stacked in a pile. Sophie was skinny and pale, white like her gown that was soon tossed on the floor. The scrub nurse and registrar painted her yellow with iodine solution, then put on the blue drapes. I tried to adjust the operating theatre lights, but they were brand new, cheap and with a life of their own. Everything we had was either new and cheap, or old – the instruments, the saws, the ventilators, the heart–lung machine, all repaired time after time. That's what we had to work with, but there was no point moaning about it.

I opened her quickly. Already the blood biochemistry was poor as her disintegrating heart gave up the ghost. Sophie was pretty close to being a ghost herself now and needed to be safely on cardiopulmonary bypass, when we could correct everything by filtering her blood. When I bisected her breast-bone I could see that there was still a substantial amount of yellow fluid and debris within the pericardium around the heart, strands of infected protein, teeming with staphylococcus, that had precipitated out of the inflammatory soup. We sucked and scraped it all out, then I put in the bypass pipes and the perfusionist started his machine. For now, Sophie was safe. It was time to assess the damage.

Her juvenile left atrium was very small, so I approached it through the right atrium then across the septum between the two. Now I had sight of the mitral valve, which looked as if it were covered in seaweed. There was an abscess in the junction between the anterior and posterior leaflets to my left, the tissue deeply eroded by the bacteria and torn, causing the valve to separate away from the wall of the heart. My first impression was that it all needed to come out, but instinctively I first started to clean away the infected gunge to see what was left, gradually cutting back to the healthy tissue that would hold stitches. The first assistant was hauling uncomfortably on the atrial retractor, bewildered as to why I wasn't making my usual rapid progress. But I'd decided to try to repair the damage and save the valve, sparing Sophie the risk of lifelong anti-coagulation that would most likely rob her of a safe pregnancy.

I wondered whether I could rebuild the damaged edges of both leaflets with pericardium. The fibrous membrane from around the heart was the most appropriate material to use, but because Sophie's own pericardium was teeming with bacteria I used cow pericardium instead, sheets of sterilised tissue that are prepared by the cardiovascular industry for the specific purpose of repairing the heart or blood vessels. I cut out an oval patch to sew into the mushy heart wall, onto which I reattached the flail valve leaflets. This resulted in the valve orifice becoming smaller, but not sufficiently to obstruct the flow. At one corner I used an extra strip of human aorta to reinforce the repair. Picasso would have been proud of me. Or perhaps Henry Moore, the sculptor. Sophie's heart now contained bits of both dead person and dead cow. I hoped this piece of applied fine art would stand up to the pressure when the heart started to pump again. We would soon find out.

Before closing up I washed the cavities of the heart carefully with saline solution. Children's hearts start up very quickly and we didn't want any infected debris in Sophie's brain. We would soon have echo pictures of the repair from the probe in her oesophagus. There were the usual microbubbles of air whizzing around inside the left ventricle, like a snow storm on the screen. I made a small puncture hole in the highest point of the aorta and they all fizzed out into the atmosphere, where they belonged.

As the heart flipped into regular rhythm we could see that the valve was competent, with just a trace of a leak – nothing more.

The time had come to think about separating from the bypass machine. This presented another challenge, but the heart was already looking better, with languid, coordinated contractions. All four valves opened and closed nicely on the echo, so I asked that it be slowly slid off from bypass. The little heart was soon on its own again, pumping away with pressure up to 100 mm Hg, and the repair was holding.

As if orchestrated to the minute, Nick Archer's balding head suddenly appeared around the door, so I asked my bespectacled registrar to close up the chest and went over to speak with him. Archer wondered why the operation had taken longer than usual and was concerned for the parents. The more intelligent the waiting relatives, the greater their insight and the higher their anxiety levels. But he was particularly pleased by the word 'repair'. Although we even had some babies with artificial mitral valves, striking a balance between inadequate and excessive anticoagulation was difficult, boiling down essentially to stroke versus bleeding. Anticoagulation was also a concern for young women who wanted babies, since warfarin can cause foetal abnormalities or bleeding into the placenta. It was difficult stuff to deal with, but now Sophie wouldn't need it. Archer took me off to meet the divorced parents, with their respective new partners. They were all huddled together for moral support, each fearing the worst.

I have no affinity with triumphalism and I never wanted to play God. But parents do crave reassurance from the man that did the job. Indeed I had once been on the other side of the fence when a member of my family had heart surgery and I ached to be told that everything was fine. So that was precisely what I told them. Yet in the back of my mind I wondered whether an abscess remained in Sophie's heart muscle, as I'd seen an unusual bulge beneath the repair in the wall of the left ventricle. I had cleaned out some pus and expected it to heal, but this staphylococcus was so bloody aggressive.

By the time I returned to the operating theatre my registrar had closed the chest and Sophie was being wheeled out. I still needed to draw the steps of the operation in her notes so that others could understand what had been done. Then, with the poor girl settled in intensive care, I went home the hero, while the complex little family took it in turns to sit by Sophie's bedside through the night, loving her towards recovery. They had hope again. Fear for the time being was dispelled.

I was back with her by 6.30 the following morning. Because we had no other children's heart surgeon in those days, no one else to take responsibility, there was no on call or off call, no day or night. It was just me if something happened. Sophie had been stable overnight and her mum was with her, grasping her hand, not about to let her go. But her temperature was high again. We had stirred up the hornets' nest and staphylococcus was angry. Billions of them. She still needed powerful vasopressor drugs to maintain an adequate blood pressure, and her kidneys had stopped producing urine.

During the morning Archer did another echo. The left ventricle was working well and the mitral valve looked good. There was the usual accumulation of blood and blood clot around the heart – there always was at this stage – but Sophie remained stable for the next forty-eight hours and was taken off the ventilator. Next day she went to the adolescent ward known as Melanie's, back to a single room. She still had that swinging temperature, and we blamed it on complement activation, my great discovery in Alabama.

4 March, 11.35 am. Crash call to Melanie's Ward. One week after her emergency surgery, and fortunately with her mother Fiona in the room, Sophie suddenly collapsed without warning. She was lying prostrate on the floor, pulseless and not breathing, when the paediatric resuscitation team burst in and started cardiac massage. The anaesthetist hand-pumped the black gas bag, inflating her lungs with oxygen. An intravenous injection of adrenaline restored a modest blood pressure, just long enough for a quick echocardiogram. This showed her pericardium to be filled with blood. The little heart was squeezed and unable to fill. Worse still, there seemed to be a hole in the heart wall where there should be muscle.

An abscess cavity had ruptured directly below the repaired valve, so my worst fear had indeed materialised. The cardiology registrar attempted to aspirate blood with a needle but it clotted off rapidly. Then she arrested again, needing more cardiac massage. The lady registrar called me in my office. I just told them to get Sophie round to theatre immediately, because if I opened her on the ward she'd die. I knew what to expect and needed to rush her back on the bypass machine. I could readily visualise the problem, and for once I was concerned that I couldn't fix it. I had that gut-wrenching feeling that she wouldn't even make it to the operating table. I hoped she would – but I didn't expect it.

With repeated boluses of adrenaline and intermittent cardiac massage, Sophie did reach theatre, and her arrival was luckily well timed between my colleague's planned operations, so God must have been sitting on her shoulder. She came directly through to the operating table, where I was scrubbed and waiting, and we hurriedly sliced through the skin stitches and snipped the wires holding the sternum together, then I unceremoniously ripped them out and ratchetted open the retractor. The heart was encased in blood clot, a purple gelatinous mass just like fresh liver that all had to be scooped out by hand so the heart could fill and eject blood again. It was beating like the clappers in response to the drugs, but then fresh blood suddenly gushed out from behind, filling the pericardium. I needed to see where it was coming from. I suspected that the abscess below the mitral valve had eroded through the wall of the ventricle, and that the muscle itself was now mush and wouldn't hold stitches. The nightmare scenario.

The anaesthetist's echo probe in her oesophagus confirmed my worst fears. There was a ragged abscess cavity that had ruptured through the ventricular wall beneath the important circumflex coronary artery. I had never seen or heard of this before in hundreds of cases of bacterial endocarditis, nor had I even read about it in the surgical journals. So this was going to have to be a 'make it up as I go along' job. One thing was certain, however. Had I implanted a rigid artificial valve first time around, that whole fragile junction between the left atrium and left ventricle would have fallen apart and been irretrievable. At least the valve repair remained intact. It was clear that I should attempt to close the abscess from outside the heart, because if I messed with my previous fix I would never get it together again. A complex conglomeration of human and cow was all that held this part of Sophie's heart together.

I slipped in the cannulas and rushed her back onto the bypass machine, intending to empty the heart before I tried to lift it. I then stopped it in a chilled, flaccid state with cardioplegia so it became still and cold like a heart on the butcher's slab. This time, when I lifted it, the bulge at the back was obvious. Bacterial enzymes had dissolved the muscle protein and the antibiotics had failed to protect it from liquefaction. As a result, the abscess had expanded. I asked for a stitch on a large needle and attempted to draw the edges of healthy muscle together.

I knew where the circumflex coronary artery should be but couldn't see it within the inflammatory morass. In went those deep stitches through what I thought was uninfected tissue around the margins of the mush. As I tied the knots I was concerned lest the suture material cheese-wire through, with fearful consequences. At this point, there was no bleeding because the heart was empty and had no pressure inside it. And, sure enough, the bulge was gone. When I let blood back into the heart it began to squirm, then contract again. But from the ECG I could see that we were in trouble. Instead of discrete spikes we had the rounded hills characteristic of heart muscle starved of blood – myocardial ischemia is the medical term. I knew that I had trapped that critical coronary artery in the stitches. A list of suitable expletives came to mind, but for everyone's sake I kept my mouth shut. Sophie couldn't survive the inevitable heart attack. I needed to take down the repair and start all over again. Battle of the Bulge, round two.

We gave more cold cardioplegia solution, then I picked up the heart and carefully cut away the stitches and replaced them with fresh ones at a different angle, this time further away from where I anticipated the coronary artery to be. Still not confident with the repair on which her life depended, I tried a belt-and-braces approach, covering the area with biological glue and a haemostatic gauze patch, just like repairing a hole in my trousers. Then we tried coming off bypass once again. This time the ECG returned to normal – pointed peaks in the Dolomites rather than the whalebacks of the Brecon Beacons. That part of the ventricle had its blood supply again. Now we needed the botch job to hold up. My operation note was prescriptive and cautious: 'Keep the blood pressure below 90 mm Hg. Keep Sophie asleep on the ventilator for seven days. It will not be possible to retrieve another catastrophe.'

As the chest was closed again, the back of the heart remained dry with no bleeding at all. The whole team felt a huge sense of relief when Sophie made it back to paediatric intensive care. The poor family were still in shock, waiting huddled together in the relatives' room and mentally disintegrating with the intolerable suspense. I explained that an abscess had eaten its way through the heart wall, that I had never seen this terrible problem before but we had done our best to fix it. Then the usual defensive crap. The next twenty-four hours would be critical. The outcome remained uncertain, but where there was life there was hope. This was all true, but it felt hollow on my tongue as I faced the three sad faces, each too stunned to ask any questions apart from when could they see her. I quietly withdrew and flipped my emotion switch to the off position.

Leaving the grief behind, I passed Archer on the corridor on his way to see Sophie. In an understated fashion he said what he always says: 'Well done, Westaby.'

I appreciated that, and subsequently learned that he wasn't expecting to see her again. Archer and the intensive care doctors took over for the night. I should have called in to apologise to my cancelled patient but I didn't. I wasn't in the mood to apologise to anyone for anything by that point. I used to lose track of time when I was operating, and by now it was 9 pm. I needed a beer and some downtime. As was often the case I couldn't sleep, expecting the phone to ring at any time. Eventually I pre-empted the call. At 3.30 in the morning I rang the unit to see how Sophie was getting on. She was stable but still had that swinging fever. They were actively cooling her and she was still not passing urine. Then the important phrase: 'There's no bleeding.' So I lapsed gratefully into unconsciousness.

Less than twelve hours after that, Sophie and I were back in theatre. Battle of the Bulge, phase three. At 1.30 pm the chest drains rapidly filled with blood and her blood pressure disappeared. Now she was bleeding to death. Again, I knew there was no point opening her in the intensive care unit as they wanted me to do. Either we let her go in peace – the logical option – or I needed her back on the bypass machine while I reconsidered the options, if there were any.

My intensive care colleagues kept squeezing in uncross-matched donor blood through the drips, managing to hold the blood pressure at around 60 mm Hg. Then we rushed her bed and overflowing chest drains down the corridor, scattering wide-eyed hospital visitors and leaving a stream of blood in our wake. Had this happened during the night there would have been no chance. Once more my great team pulled together and we got her onto the operating table before she completely exsanguinated.

Her sternum was open again in minutes, the chest full of fresh blood and clot compressing the heart. Bags of O negative blood were still being squeezed in through her neck veins, but within minutes we were back on cardio-pulmonary bypass for the third time, albeit with a sense of resignation. Thinking, 'What the hell do we do now?', we had pulled back from the brink again – to what end? We had to draw the line somewhere, but not yet. As Albert

Camus wrote, 'Where there is no hope, it is incumbent upon us to invent it.' The bottom line was that Sophie was only fifteen.

I was gripped by a fierce determination to get her through, but doing it by the book was not going to work here. Grim Reaper was outmanoeuvring me with my conventional approach. If this infected muscle was ever going to heal, it simply couldn't happen while the left ventricle was continuously generating pressure and supporting the circulation, as it was the relentless pressure swings within the chamber that was causing it to rupture. This time Sophie had started to bleed when her sedation wore off. Her conscious state lightened, her anxiety rose, so her blood pressure shot up. Then whoosh. Torn muscle, followed by cardiac tamponade.

She needed a new heart, but that was not possible. Her desolate mother would have gladly given hers, but even if we'd had an organ donor in the adjacent theatre no one would contemplate a transplant in an infected child. No one except me, that is, but we could never find a heart in time, unless I commandeered one from a philanthropic medical student … Then suddenly, amid the panic and delirious fantasy, the penny dropped. My only practical option was to actively empty the left side of the heart and keep it empty. That would remove all the pressure from within the chamber. I could use a left ventricular assist device (LVAD) to suck down the left ventricle, maintain the circulation and rest the damaged muscle while antibiotics dealt with the infection. This might enable it to heal. Had the technology ever been used for this purpose before? Absolutely not. But that was even more reason for me to give it a try. In the highly unlikely scenario of it proving successful, I could publish a paper about it.

I was then reminded that we no longer had a Levitronix pump as my charitable funds had run out and we had used the last one recently on the baby. To my knowledge we didn't have any more lifesaving equipment, and in the mortality statistics only one individual would carry the can for this death – me. The blame-and-shame system we worked in would record this one as a death after mitral valve repair. Lifesaving equipment is expensive but death is cheap. Push mortality rates into the public arena, but don't give the stroppy surgeons the tools to do the job. Pause for a moment to reflect on the morality of that.

Then Brian the perfusionist came to my rescue. He had a different type of centrifugal blood pump on trial in one of our heart–lung machines. It was said to be safe to use continuously for three weeks at a time, unlike the conventional roller pump, where three hours was too long. I felt that three weeks would be sufficient – inflammatory adhesions and fibrous scar ought to plug the hole in that time. We should go for it since there were no other options.

While the perfusion team assembled the equipment, I stopped Sophie's heart for the very last time and searched for the rent in the ventricular wall. Luckily it was on the edge of the infamous bulge, well away from that coronary artery. The stitches had cheese-wired through the fragile muscle again, so with more stitches and much more expensive tissue glue I stuck the back of the heart to the fibrous pericardium, using every possible trick to lessen the risk of further catastrophe because the next exsanguination would undoubtedly be her last.

This Rotaflow pump was very simple – there was just one knob to boost the flow or turn it down – and I emptied out the left ventricle by sucking blood from its apex through a wide-bore cannula, with the tubing that connected to the external pump circuit emerging from below Sophie's ribs. Through a second tube the pump returned this blood to the aorta. Bleeding was still going to be our biggest problem; after three cardiopulmonary bypass runs within a short period of time, Sophie's blood wouldn't clot, so we needed masses of donor clotting factors and yet more blood transfusion. The perfusionist started the whirling rotary pump at its lowest speed, aiming to transfer gradually from the one extracorporeal circuit to the next. Once more there would be no pulse pressure on the monitors, just the average pressure of the continuous, non-pulsatile blood flow. Meanwhile the wounded left ventricle was still contracting but not pumping, while the right ventricle continued to push blood through the lungs. Magic. So far, so good. We had renewed grounds for hope.

Because of the coagulation problems and diffuse bleeding, I decided to leave Sophie's sternum wide open for forty-eight hours. We packed swabs around the heart, placed an adhesive plastic drape over the chest, and drainage tubes were brought out alongside the assist device cannulas. With tubes emerging from everywhere it was a terrifying spectacle for the family, and was also a little too much for the paediatric intensive care unit this time. We took her back to adult intensive care, where our senior nurses had more experience with pulseless patients and where the parents of other sick children wouldn't be spooked by the sight.

As the bleeding damped down, Sophie remained stable. Both her kidneys and her liver had taken a hit, but dialysis could cope with that. Mum Fiona stayed remarkably calm, although the gore took its toll – it was a terrible strain for Sophie's poor sister, who stayed away from school. Two days later we removed the blood-soaked packs and closed the chest over the hardware to reduce the risk of further infection. By now the blood was clotting, the oozing had stopped and the front of the heart looked fine. I was definitely not going to explore the back. The pump was working well and I was determined to leave it in place for at least another ten days to give the abscess site the best chance to heal. In the meantime, we learned that the mighty staphylococcus was resistant to our second combination of antibiotics, so we changed the drugs again. At last the high temperature abated.

Sophie was kept heavily sedated on the ventilator for three weeks, which helped to keep her blood pressure under control. Then the dreaded fungus candida crept in under the radar. We discovered it first in the urinary tract, where it could prove life threatening if we were unable to control it. Now the so-called period of stability was turning into a nightmare, so we felt it was time to initiate some forward movement to reduce the risk of more complications. The pump was doing its job splendidly and it was time to let her wake up.

When the sedation was switched off, Sophie woke up promptly and responded to her parents. With awareness came higher blood pressure, which we could control, and there was still no bleeding. The poor lass was clearly terrified by her plight, and I suspected that there were signs of brain injury. We tried to explain why she had pipes full of rushing blood coming out of her belly, assuring her that she was safe and that we would shortly remove them. Soon afterwards the nurses noticed that she was not moving her left arm or leg – they were paralysed and didn't respond to pain. Either infected material or blood clot from the damaged heart wall had found its way up the arteries to her brain. She was paralysed at fifteen. Why did we deserve that?

This was devastating for her parents, and the Battle of the Bulge was now beginning to take its toll on me. Why would anyone want to do this job, day after day, night after night? Healed heart, buggered brain was not what I had hoped for.

The following day I took Sophie back to the operating theatre to remove the cannulas from the left ventricle and aorta. I was delighted to find that there was no clot in the centrifugal pump or the rest of the system and that Sophie's heart looked great on echo, apart from a residual crater beneath the mitral valve, which was now a blind-ended pouch. Miraculously, after all the cardiac massage and surgery, the repaired valve had held up and was still functioning well. I gave the chest and pericardium a good washout with antiseptic solution, while once again assiduously avoiding the back of the heart. Then we closed her up for the last time. This was the end of Sophie's marathon surgery, the final phase of a long, bloody battle of relentless attrition. We had succeeded in keeping her alive, but at what cost?

For the family's sake it was important to stay positive as they were all shell-shocked. Mother Fiona had witnessed all three resuscitation attempts, each time enduring the agonising wait to see if Sophie would come out of theatre to intensive care or to the mortuary, dressed in her white hospital gown or wrapped in a shroud. Right now it was Westaby 3, Grim Reaper 0. Did we have a plan to keep it that way? There was absolutely no precedent. It was a unique case.

As I saw it we needed to do two things. First, continue to screw down the blood pressure, with Sophie's own heart supporting the circulation. Second, keep her brain well supplied with oxygen to minimise cerebral damage. The brain possesses more resilience than most people expect, and the majority of strokes recover substantially, with improvement more likely in a young person. This was the positive message that both the nurses and family needed to hear. They all needed some hope that she wouldn't be bedridden for what remained of her life.

After considering the options, I decided to play safe by insisting that Sophie stay asleep on the ventilator for another two weeks. We would only move her for a brain scan when I was satisfied that we could do so without risk. In the meantime she was still not passing urine and needed continuous kidney dialysis. Kidneys don't like sepsis and low blood pressure, but they always recover.

With the hardware out, it was time to move her back to paediatric intensive care, a smaller unit with a more consistent nursing team and mercifully more peaceful nights.

Sophie's brain scan showed several small areas of focal damage with swelling around them. These were probably caused by embolisation of infected debris from the heart, and it was important to try to prevent them turning into cerebral abscesses. She would be kept on the intravenous antibiotics regime for another six weeks, which is routine for endocarditis, and the inflammatory swelling around the damaged areas would undoubtedly disappear. Would Sophie remain paralysed? We received the standard answer from the neurologists – they hoped she wouldn't but only time would tell.

On 1 April, the day of fools, Sophie's sedation was finally withdrawn and she woke up promptly. She could breathe well enough and respond to commands, so we proceeded to remove the tube from her throat and raise the bed head. Mum and Dad sat on either side, holding her hands. When Dad squeezed Sophie's left hand she responded with weak but unequivocal movement. But she was obviously having difficulty in finding words and articulating sentences – the brain scan had predicted this, showing a small but strategic defect in the speech area. There was light at the end of the tunnel. Her attempts to communicate definitely made sense, and my job was done.

Brain recovery is always slow. Sophie would need ongoing care from nurses, physiotherapists, occupational therapists and a host of different medical staff. They all pulled together to move her forward, then the community services rallied round. Over the following months the paralysis and speech impediment got better, then she went back to school and eventually on to college, with her considerable intellect intact. Against all the odds, Sophie survived. Even I find it difficult to understand how we succeeded over those weeks. Divine help, I suspect. And that piece of kit on loan, more charity-shop healthcare.

I wrote a case report about the rescue technique of emptying an injured left ventricle with an assist device and it was published in an erudite American journal so that others might use the method in desperation. Sophie's case illustrated the very best of NHS hospital team work and the triumph of hope over misery. So many dedicated staff worked way beyond their prescribed hours in the struggle to save her. Ironically, our pioneering efforts were questioned every step of the way and they generated huge costs for the hospital. But what is healthcare there for? Ten years on, I still see Sophie and her family socially. On the tenth anniversary of the Battle of the Bulge we had dinner at Fiona's Oxford college, Lady Margaret's Hall, together with the eminent brain surgeon and author Henry Marsh. Heart surgeons and brain surgeons are very different, but we agreed on one thing. Life is precious. It was great to see an animated Sophie holding her own in that rarefied academic environment.

10

resilience

23 October 2009

NHS CONSENT FORM 2

Parental Agreement to Investigation or Treatment for a Child or Young Person

NHS organisation: John Radcliffe Hospital, Oxford

Patient's name: Oliver Walker

Date of birth: 11 February 2003

Name of proposed procedure or course of treatment:
Excision of Cor Triatriatum membrane – salvage procedure

Statement of health professional

The intended benefits: to sustain life – at present death is inevitable without surgery.

Serious or frequently occurring risks: surgical mortality, at least 30%, bleeding, the damaging effects of cardiopulmonary bypass, need for reoperation.

Other procedures: blood transfusion, echocardiography.

I handed the form to Richard, Oliver's trembling father. His mother Nicky was already in meltdown. She was watching her son die from a rare congenital heart condition that had taken the NHS six years to diagnose. Not in the Highlands of Scotland or far-flung west Wales. Not even in Scunthorpe, but in central London. Easy for me to criticise, since I never have to make a diagnosis – the cardiologists do that for me, I'm just the plumber. But one thing I did understand by then was always listen to the mother, because no one knows her child better. If Mum insists there is something seriously wrong, you can bet your life there will be.

For Nicky it had been a long, hard grind to persuade the doctors. Now, years later, a flash Harry of a surgeon who had just walked in from Heathrow Airport was pushing her son down the corridor to the operating theatres as fast as the bed, ventilator, drips and drains would move. We were that close to losing him to something he had been born with, a bog-standard congenital heart condition.

Oliver had been delivered at St Mary's Hospital, Paddington, one of our great London teaching hospitals, in the same maternity unit where our royals choose to have their babies. It was a normal but noisy birth, and Oliver appeared to be pink and robust. His heart rate was a little rapid, but after the shock of being squeezed through a greasy rabbit hole into the cold world, no one at the hospital thought anything of it. Nicky said he didn't feed at all well – tugging on her nipples made him breathless and agitated – but he wasn't a 'blue baby', just very chesty. So damned chesty and breathless, in fact, that the little family were in and out of St Mary's on a regular basis, as if it were a football ground and they had season tickets. It seemed that any cough or cold could become life-threatening.

Eventually it became embarrassing for them, a case of the 'not you again' syndrome, and in the casualty department they were known as 'frequent fliers'. Yet St Mary's was a top hospital and this was a family who were deeply concerned for their child. Nicky grew paranoid about being labelled a neurotic mother who couldn't cope, because on many occasions they were sent away from the hospital or general practice having been told that the boy was fine and there was nothing wrong with him. So often did they return in distress that Oliver was investigated repeatedly, with many distressing attempts to draw blood, then frequent X-rays so that he almost glowed in the dark. Every conceivable lung condition was considered: bronchiolitis, cystic fibrosis and pneumonia, on numerous occasions. Sure, his little lungs sounded congested, but nothing came up positive. They considered a stomach hernia with gastro-oesophageal reflux and inhalation of his gastric contents. He didn't have that either. There was nothing to find, yet he was constantly struggling for breath.

Oliver now had a younger brother two years his junior. The fact that he couldn't keep up with him caused Oliver extreme frustration. There was a twenty-minute walk to his primary school, which a four-year-old should be able to manage. Yet two-year-old Charlie would often climb out of the buggy and walk, which allowed 'lazy' Oliver to sit down and be pushed to school. Clearly that wasn't right. Others could see that there was a problem, but the doctors had no answer. What causes breathlessness at the slightest provocation, failure to thrive and perpetual lack of energy? A boy who couldn't play football with his friends or walk to the park, who sat in the corner looking dejected at birthday parties? This was all heartbreaking for Nicky. But however many times she was brushed aside by the medical profession, she couldn't possibly give up, and I greatly admired her for this.

Eventually Oliver was referred to the chest physicians at the Royal Brompton Hospital. There was nowhere to go after that. It was the National Heart and Lung Institute, and they said that the only things that could cause his symptoms were his heart or lungs – but his lungs were normal and his heart was not enlarged on the chest X-ray, ostensibly ruling out the usual causes of heart failure in children. So goodbye again, even from this world-famous hospital.

Soon Nicky was on the phone once more, pleading for her poor boy's life. They must have missed something. Oliver simply couldn't run or play with the other kids at school. The teachers had remarked upon it, other mothers could see it. Sure, he looked normal sitting in front of the doctor, but that was all he could do. Just sit. So the Brompton doctors decided to watch him run up and down the hospital corridor, then checked his heart rate – he couldn't manage to complete this easy exercise test and his heart rate went through the roof even after a few steps.

With such negligible exercise tolerance there simply had to be something wrong.

Now they really did have to look inside the heart. With the stethoscope, the valves sounded fine but perhaps quieter than they should have been – lub, the mitral valve closes; dub, the aortic valve closes – but the heart rate was so fast that it was impossible to detect a murmur. That was Friday. Concerned that there must be something seriously wrong with his heart, Nicky was asked to bring Oliver back yet again on Monday for an echocardiogram. This would define the anatomy in detail and incorporate an ECG to detect any heart rhythm problem. Because the valves sounded normal and the left ventricle appeared small on the X-ray, Nicky hoped that nothing serious would be found. She arranged to meet her sister for lunch in Chelsea after the tests, as a treat for her son.

By now Oliver was used to hospitals. Moreover, he had been reassured that there would be no needles this time, just sticky jelly on his chest and a slippery probe sliding around. He lay perfectly still on the couch while the young lady echocardiographer watched the images flashing on the screen and chatted away cheerfully to Nicky. All seemed relaxed and normal until the lady stopped moving the probe and suddenly went quiet, her gaze fixed. In the space of an instant her expression changed from unconcerned to dumbfounded.

'What is it?' asked an alarmed Nicky, but there was no response.

The girl was mesmerised by an abnormality on the screen, but had no idea what she was looking at. On the third time of asking, she heard the tone of desperation in Nicky's voice. All she could say was, 'Oh I'm sorry, I need to fetch the consultant.' Oliver lay there oblivious to the sudden air of panic, while Nicky's circulation was flooded with adrenaline and she started to have a panic attack. She felt the urge to call her husband at work but had nothing to tell him yet, except that the woman had found something terrible inside Oliver's heart. It had to be terrible, otherwise she wouldn't have rushed off like that.

For six long years Nicky had been sure that there was something seriously wrong with Oliver but had always been relieved when told she was mistaken. Not any more, although at least the consultant was calm. He returned the echo probe to Oliver's bony chest and started to work back through the images. The right atrium was mildly dilated, the right ventricle thickened and the pulmonary artery dilated, none of which had been picked up on the many chest X-rays. Put together, this suggested that there was some sort of obstruction to the blood flow through Oliver's lungs. What's more, the left atrium was dilated, while the left ventricle seemed small and underfilled. This would normally suggest narrowing of the mitral valve, as in patients with rheumatic fever, but the mitral valve leaflets looked thin and normal.

The experienced consultant knew precisely what he was looking at, yet the condition was so exceptionally rare that this was the first time he had diagnosed it himself. Inaudibly he muttered, 'Cor triatriatum, that explains it!', although that left neither Nicky nor the echocardiographer any the wiser. Blood was swirling

around within the left atrium but not filling the left ventricle in the way that it should. Why? Because there was a
thin membrane obstructing the left atrium and all four
veins from the lungs, so blood couldn't get to the orifice
of the mitral valve. The only way through was a tiny aperture 3 mm in diameter, contrasting starkly with the normal
mitral valve orifice of 18 mm for a six-year-old boy.

Cor triatriatum translates from the Latin as 'heart with
three atrial chambers'. Oliver's blood was dammed up
behind the obstruction, causing congestion in otherwise
normal lungs, so there was no way that he could increase
blood flow to his body while exerting himself because his
entire cardiac output had to squeeze through the restric-
tion. All of Oliver's symptoms were caused by this
congenital anomaly. His very existence had been a nightmare of untold physical and psychological misery, while
his poor parents had been sent away time after time with
misinformation. But at least he was still alive. For now,
that is.

The paediatric cardiologist was justifiably shocked by
the severity of the blockage and immediately called a
surgical colleague. Oliver had suffered quite long enough
and needed that membrane removed as a matter of
urgency. In the meantime, poor Nicky had disintegrated.
Richard was at work, waiting for news. She managed to
dial his mobile number but was too emotional to articu-
late the problem or explain that Oliver needed open heart
surgery as soon as possible. The kind cardiologist tried to
put things in perspective for Richard, telling him that at
least they had finally identified the problem. Although it

was rare, there were experienced cardiac surgeons at the hospital who would deal with it at low risk. Rare did not necessarily mean difficult, then after the surgery Oliver should catch up and have a normal life. Nicky's sister came to the Brompton to support her, and everyone headed home to take it all in. But they had now moved house some distance away from central London, to Beaconsfield.

Oliver went back to school the following morning, his parents trying to maintain a semblance of routine before the operation. The teachers were warned of his situation. Suddenly he had a serious heart condition, which explained why he couldn't keep up with the other kids. Some felt guilty for the things they had said about him, others because they had tried to push him too hard. Children with congenital heart disease often suffer like this. They have two arms and two legs, but their engine doesn't work. They are the blue kids who squat in the playground to relieve their breathlessness. Other kids poke fun at them and they always come last on sports day. Their parents burn up inside, but try to smile and keep things normal for them.

21 October 2009. I was giving a talk about ventricular assist devices at the European Society of Cardiothoracic Surgeons in Vienna, so there was no children's heart surgeon back in Oxford. Meanwhile Nicky was at home in Beaconsfield, trying to get her three children ready for school. Two of them were looking after themselves, but poor Oliver had a barking cough and couldn't get out of bed. With a temperature exceeding 38°C, he was already

panting for breath with an imperceptibly rapid heart rate, and his skin had turned yellow.

In a panic, Nicky bundled all three children into the car and was already waiting at the medical centre when the doctors arrived. There was no crass reassurance or chastisement this time, and an ambulance was called immediately. This took Oliver and his mother directly to the nearest hospital, Stoke Mandeville on the outskirts of Aylesbury, while the bemused brothers, half-dressed, had to wait at the doctors' surgery for family friends to pick them up and take them to school.

During the winter of 2009 there was an epidemic of swine flu in Britain, and several cases had been identified at Oliver's school. The H1N1 virus belongs to the influenza family and is generally found in the respiratory tract of pigs. With an incubation period of as little as twenty-four hours, the strain responsible for the epidemic had been imported from Mexico and was highly contagious. It inflicted a mortality rate of 5 per cent, principally by causing pneumonia in the elderly or vulnerable. Oliver was nothing if not vulnerable.

At Stoke Mandeville he was taken directly to an isolation room, not the general children's ward. The swine flu diagnosis proved correct, yet there was no immediate therapeutic option to make the virulent viral infection any better – when Oliver complained of headache with photophobia then coughed up blood, his doctors wanted to give him the antiviral agent zanamivir, better known by its brand name Relenza, directly into the blood stream, but there wasn't any in the hospital. By the evening the poor boy was desperately ill, suffering from two rare conditions that were conspiring to kill him. Given that Nicky stayed with him minute after minute, perhaps the best description of the next few hours comes from her letter to me several years later:

> It is hard to convey the horror you feel as you face losing a child. I love all my children equally but had a special bond with Oliver through the sheer number of hours and days we spent together in hospital over his first six years of life. During that night in Stoke Mandeville, Oliver was becoming increasingly restless and uncomfortable. He was leaning up against me in bed, then he said, 'Mummy, I can't breathe any more,' at which point I screamed for help. After that I can only describe it as all hell breaking loose. Alarms started ringing, someone forced a pipe down his throat, then someone else cut off his pyjamas to shove a drip cannula into his groin. I was bundled out of the room in a state of shock. Some kind mother from the children's ward came to hold me until I was allowed back into the room. I was truly terrified.

Curiously, Oliver hadn't even been connected to a mechanical ventilator. A doctor and a male nurse knelt beside him all through the night and manually pumped oxygen into his lungs through a black Ambu bag. Perhaps there were no children's intensive care beds there, or none available, but the two kept Oliver alive until the paediatric intensive care retrieval team arrived from Oxford.

Only then was he attached to a respirator for the return journey in the ambulance.

Because of the swine flu, Oliver was housed in an isolation room with full monitoring of his cardiovascular status via cannulas in both arteries and veins. None of the readings were encouraging. He had very low oxygen levels in the blood, low blood pressure, a dangerously fast heart rate and his kidneys were not producing urine. Skilled manipulation of vasopressor drugs and diuretics improved the situation for a while, but any conventional lines of treatment were hindered by the blockage within the heart. Because of the obstructive physiology, there was no means of relieving the severe congestion in Oliver's lungs and liver, nor any method to increase the blood flow around his body. With progressive jaundice and kidney failure, the metabolic mayhem in his blood stream worsened by the minute.

That Thursday evening I had dinner in a fancy restaurant in Vienna, while Nick Archer was on a flight back from Australia, neither of us of any use to Oliver or his anxious family. Fortunately, there was a very conscientious locum cardiologist on call, Dr Dimitrescu from Slovenia, and the intensive care doctors asked her whether she could do anything to help. It was blatantly obvious to her that Oliver's unique combination of conditions would prove fatal if nothing changed, so she promptly called the surgeons at the Brompton. They offered to operate on the boy the following week, as long as the viral illness was under control. Toxic infections alongside cardiovascular collapse and liver and kidney failure did not provide the ideal circumstances for a spin on the heart–lung machine.

By 2009 all cardiac centres were under scrutiny regarding their death rates, the days of salvage surgery having passed. What's more, the Royal Brompton was a heart and lung centre with no specialists in general paediatrics. They were less well equipped to deal with the infectious illness, while the Oxford intensive care doctors were better placed to manage the dire consequences of swine flu. To do that they gave sildenefil – or Viagra, as it's better known – to reduce the blood pressure in Oliver's lung arteries, together with the antiviral drug Tamiflu, and he gradually stabilised overnight.

As the hours ticked by, Nicky was reassured to be in a dedicated children's hospital within the sprawling John Radcliffe campus. There were eight other children on ventilators, each surrounded by loving and anxious parents. The doctors seemed confident and the nurses were kind. Yet there were terrible things to be seen: the toddler with meningitis and gangrenous legs who was constantly hooked up to a kidney dialysis machine, the septic baby with a hydrocephalus who was scheduled for brain surgery, and the boy with black eyes, a bandaged head, pins in his legs and drains in his chest following a road accident. And there were a couple of my patients recovering slowly.

In the parents' sitting room each mother had her own story to tell, while over in the nurses' coffee room the doctors and nurses huddled together, exchanging details about their patients. It would be easy to become institutionalised here, but after the weekend Oliver was going to be transferred to the Brompton for his critical operation. At least that was the plan. Some of the parents asked why the risk of moving him to London was being taken when he could have his surgery here in Oxford; Nicky and Richard wondered about this too, but they had been given a definite plan and knew the Brompton well, having spent many hours there focused on Oliver's lungs while remaining totally in the dark about cor triatriatum. No one seemed to understand that term, even now.

On Friday morning Nick Archer flew in to Heathrow from Australia and I came back from Vienna. During the intensive care round, Oliver's chest X-ray was carefully scrutinised. If anything, his lungs were now less congested after the Viagra, and the diuretic drugs had boosted his urine output. On the negative side, there was a sizeable collection of free pleural fluid around the left lung – what we call a pleural effusion. If this continued to accumulate it would interfere with the ventilation of the lung and predispose him to pneumonia. The consensus was that the fluid should be drained, but there was too much for a simple needle aspiration. Oliver needed a proper chest drain to be inserted between his ribs. The duty registrar was designated to insert the tube, which would be done through a small incision beneath the left armpit – a routine procedure, particularly in any heart surgery unit. Sedated and unconscious, Oliver would know nothing about it. The procedure appeared to go well, since 400 ml of straw-coloured fluid deposited itself rapidly into the drainage bottle. Job done.

Archer being Archer, he called into the hospital on his way home from Heathrow. Dr Dimitrescu was pleased to see him back, having wanted some moral support with Oliver's care over the weekend. By then, Nicky felt emotionally drained:

> I had my other two sons visiting that afternoon because it was half term. I had left Oliver looked after by a gowned and masked nurse so I could show the boys where Mum and Dad were staying in the parents' accommodation. The phone rang in the room and a nurse just told me to get back to the unit immediately. I knew something was terribly wrong. I had left him with just one nurse and came back to a room full of people, none of whom had bothered to mask up. One of them was Dr Archer. Since inserting the chest drain, Oliver's blood pressure had drifted down, then disappeared altogether. Once the chest tube had drained the clear fluid, a small amount of bright red blood came out, then nothing. Amid the frantic efforts to resuscitate him they had called for a chest X-ray. Dr Archer was staring at it on the screen. The left chest cavity was now completely opaque – what they called a 'white out'.

Insertion of the chest drain had either torn an intercostal artery, which runs in a groove below the rib, or penetrated the lung itself. Either way, the outcome was the same: a left chest full of blood and no blood pressure in the circulation. So why didn't blood come out of the drain itself? Because fresh blood clots rapidly and blood clot had occluded the child-sized drainage tube – hence a trickle of fresh blood, then nothing. After that the ongoing bleeding silently filled poor Oliver's chest. Initially the circulation compensates by constricting the peripheral small arteries, but eventually the whole system decompensates and the shit hits the fan. This could well be the end of the road.

Archer had two instructions: first, 'Give him some uncrossmatched blood fast'; second, 'Find out whether Westaby is back in the country.' The switchboard put out a call for me during the Friday afternoon rush hour. I had just turned off the Oxford ring road heading for Woodstock and was looking forward to seeing my family. The operator told me that I was needed in the paediatric intensive care unit right away. I asked what for, assuming that something had gone wrong with one of my babies.

She just said, 'Sorry, but Dr Archer wants you there.'

No point trying to debate that, so I headed back to the hospital as fast as I could, deposited my car in an ambulance bay and purposefully strode down the corridor to paediatric intensive care. I didn't need to ask which patient they wanted me to see. The isolation room was packed with doctors and nurses, all with grim expressions on their faces. I could hear a woman weeping in the relatives' room. So much so that I feared I was too late. There was none of the usual banter, no 'What kept you, Westaby?' that would normally greet me when I had broken my neck to drive into town in record time. The gravity of the moment told the story.

Oliver had no perceptible blood pressure and a heart rate so rapid that it was not achieving anything of significance. The paediatric registrar was squeezing a bag of blood, forcing it into Oliver as fast as it would transit his constricted veins. Nick showed me the chest X-ray and summarised the case: 'He has cor triatriatum with an obstructed left heart and has just filled his left pleural cavity with blood. On top of that he has swine flu. He's going to die in the next few minutes unless you can get him onto the heart–lung machine.' So not exactly, 'Welcome back. How was the conference?'

I went to the parents' room with that consent form already filled in and my section signed. I apologised that there was no time for introductions or explanations. Oliver was close to death and we had to move fast. I needed to be pushing the bed down the corridor, not bullshitting about risks and benefits.

This was poor Nicky's written record of the conversation:

I remember saying that we didn't want him to have surgery as we had been told that he was too weak to operate on. You told us we had no choice. I remember your manner with us so vividly. Your confidence, reassurance and total conviction that you could help us was the only reason I let my boy go. I can't overemphasise enough how much that helped us at that awful time. Can you imagine if someone had come in, saying that they would give it a go, but things weren't looking good? You said to me as you

wheeled Oliver away that you would bring him back
to us. Then Richard and I just sat in the waiting room
holding each other, trying to work out if enough time
had gone by for him to have at least survived getting
on to the heart–lung machine.

This was generous feedback received many years later,
and very welcome too because it endorsed my disinhibited approach. Who needs introspection and equivocation
when your child is dying? The GMC might not have
endorsed my consent process, but was I troubled by that?
Draw your own conclusions. We had Oliver supine on the
operating table within five minutes of leaving intensive
care. Our paediatric cardiac anaesthetist Kate Grebenik
was not on call, but she abandoned cake-making with her
daughter to rush back into the hospital and join in the
resuscitation efforts. No questions, no ifs, no buts.

How long does it take to expose the heart in an emergency? Around one minute. Run the scalpel hard down
through both skin and fat, then run the power saw up the
bone. Prise the sternum open with the metal retractor, slit
open the fibrous pericardium and there it is. Place a couple
of purse-string stitches in the aorta and right atrium, push
in the cannulas and go 'on bypass'. Then everyone can
relax and take stock. Oliver was safe at last.

The first task now was to cut into the pleural cavity
under the left half of the breast-bone and suck out liquid
blood into the extracorporeal circuit – everything that
was transfusable we needed to put back into the blood
stream. Some of it had already clotted, slithering out like

slices of liver at the butcher's but destined for the waste bin not the frying pan. Given the metabolic derangement of near death, the anaesthetist's job was to neutralise lactic acid with sodium bicarbonate and adjust the level of potassium in the blood. In the meantime I set about stopping the heart with icy-cold cardioplegia fluid and opening the dilated part of the left atrium. With a retractor in place, the mitral valve usually comes into view immediately, but not in this curious heart. The valve itself was completely obscured by what looked like normal atrial wall. The only clue to the existence of the murderous membrane was the desperately small aperture between the main left atrial chamber and the small antechamber directly proximal to the mitral valve itself. It was like exploring Tutankhamun's tomb. One slip, and something of great importance could be damaged.

I gently inserted a right-angled forcep through the orifice and tentatively tugged on it. This didn't shift the flaccid left ventricle, so I knew I was not pulling on the mitral valve itself. Reassured, I cut through the tented membrane with scissors, revealing the valve orifice beneath. Once safe, I cut circumferentially around the whole thing, changing Oliver's outlook at a stroke – with a normal heart, swine flu wouldn't kill him. I asked our scrub nurse to put the postage-stamp-sized piece of tissue in a pot of saline solution so I could triumphantly present the trophy to the petrified parents.

The tense atmosphere in theatre lifted palpably as I sewed up the atrium, not least because the staff could see an end to the evening's dramatic proceedings. With blood flowing briskly through Oliver's tiny coronary arteries, his grateful heart muscle stiffened and started to beat spontaneously. As we allowed the left ventricle to fill, a vigorous pulse pressure wave appeared on the oscilloscope screen. Much greater volume was now pushed out into the aorta with a slower heart rate. This was the sort of instant cure that only heart surgery can offer.

Here is the penultimate paragraph of Nicky's emotional recollections from that evening:

> I think Professor said it would be three to four hours before we would hear anything. After about two hours I prised myself away from Richard and left the parents' room to find a loo. I will never forget that dim hospital corridor, empty at night, when I saw you leave the theatre and walk towards me from the other end. It seemed like forever until you got to me and I froze. I was a poleaxed, perspiring pillar of anxiety. What were you about to tell me? Was he dead or alive? I desperately tried to read your expression but the light was so poor and you were in the shadows. It was sort of in slow motion as we met face to face in that endless fateful corridor. You put your hands on my shoulders and said to me, 'It's all good, it's all good.' How I didn't just collapse in a heap I will never know! I still can't think about that moment without a tear. I have never known fear like that (well, only once before, when we were held hostage in our own home by a knifeman in a balaclava). It was a physical pain in my stomach. I still can't believe how

the stars aligned that Friday afternoon to keep Oliver here with us. It felt like you came, sprinkled some magic, then left again. You should feel proud.

Once we had corrected the biochemistry of death, removed the murderous membrane and transfused Oliver with donor blood, he never looked back. The swine flu that precipitated his sudden decline simply went away, as viruses do. The lad recovered and felt like a tight collar had been removed from his neck. He is now a normal athletic teenager, having been a whisker away from the grave. Nicky was correct about one thing. They had been in the right place at the right time – a children's hospital that could cope with his complex issues, with a dedicated team who had complete disregard for the fact they were not on call that Friday evening. What mattered to them was saving the boy's life, which they did and were thrilled about. They could all go home for the weekend and let everyone know that they had saved a young child.

Somewhat shell-shocked, I drove off towards the sunset over Woodstock. Saving Oliver had been a gargantuan effort by dedicated medical professionals, but I'd learned in Vienna that Oxford children's heart surgery was soon to be closed down. After the notorious Bristol heart scandal, a surgeon working single-handedly could never be regarded as acceptable.

Bristol was a wake-up call for my whole profession, not that there were many children's heart surgeons in the first place. The fallout made national headline news for weeks on end. Bereaved parents demonstrated in the streets, flowers were piled high outside the hospital gates as if it were a graveyard, the surgeons were vilified and made out to be mass murderers. Why? Because the death rates after heart surgery for children at the Bristol Royal Infirmary were double those in other centres, and for some operations the mortality rate was said to be prohibitively high.

The paediatric cardiologists, anaesthetists and nurses had all suspected the problem, then one broke cover. Yet there had never been an attempt to disguise the results. As the leader of the public inquiry plainly stated, 'Bristol was awash with data.' Every hospital that operated on children's hearts collected information on death rates, and the Royal College of Surgeons and the Society of Cardiothoracic Surgeons were meant to review that information.

The inquiry emphasised that Bristol had fallen victim to more general failings in the NHS. The heart specialists were split between two sites – the paediatric cardiologists in one hospital, the surgical teams in another – there were no specific children's intensive care beds, too few children's trained nurses, the critical care was 'highly disorganised', and too many facilities and too much vital equipment were reliant upon charitable donations. The report repeatedly referred to lack of funding and a blindness to the fact that this could endanger children's lives.

Both children's heart surgeons and the hospital chief executive were struck off the medical register. Then followed a public witch hunt to rein in the powerful medical profession. The inquiry concluded that the public should be informed of surgeons' death rates. Years later we are suffering the consequences – now more than 60 per cent of children's heart surgeons in the UK are overseas graduates and it is becoming progressively more difficult to fill training posts with satisfactory candidates.

Soon after Bristol, the Department of Health planned significant cuts to the number of children's heart surgery units. As Oxford was the smallest centre, I immediately knew that it would be targeted for closure. We didn't have to wait long for the onslaught. Others saw the opportunity to feed surgeons' results to the media as shrewd business. Staff at the Dr Foster Unit at Imperial College London were in the vanguard of this approach. They provided newspapers with information about topical healthcare issues in return for a fee. In 2004 the *British Medical Journal* published a paper from Dr Foster on deaths after children's heart surgery. The information had been extracted from the notoriously unreliable NHS Hospital Episode Statistics drawn together by clerical staff and used in the Bristol inquiry. Fortunately, by then the thirteen existing children's heart hospitals had begun to collect and cross-validate their own results, then submit them annually to the Central Cardiac Audit Database (CCAD).

The Dr Foster paper reported that Oxford had significantly higher death rates for children under one year of age who were operated on using the heart–lung machine. At the same time, we were accredited with the lowest mortality for babies who underwent non-bypass operations. Everyone knew that Hospital Episode Statistics were hopelessly inaccurate at the time, but now we were obliged to prove it. Oxford demanded an independent inquiry to review their allegations.

What was found cast doubt on any previous investigation from that data source. When compared with the independently validated CCAD database, Hospital Episode Statistics had missed between 5 to 147 operations for each centre and, incredibly, failed to record between 0 per cent to 73 per cent of the deaths. It happened that Oxford's data, compiled by Drs Archer and Wilson, was so accurate that every single death was included. We were the 0 per cent. In four of the largest centres, between 44 per cent to 70 per cent of the deaths were omitted! As a result, Dr Foster had claimed that the average death rate for all centres was 4 per cent, when it was double that. Because Oxford had the fewest operations and the most accurate data reporting, our mortality artificially appeared worse than other centres. In fact, we were bang in the middle of the range. The investigation concluded that Dr Foster had failed to present accurate numbers of operations, let alone death rates for most centres. What they did was to place potentially harmful conclusions in the public arena.

At this point you might be thinking that heart surgery on babies is difficult enough without having to put up with crap from grandstanders who wouldn't be allowed to change a baby's nappy. How many of the other centres were performing the infant Ross procedure? How many would have saved Sophie and Oliver? Who else had the

likes of Neil Wilson dilating aortic valves in the foetus?
That episode should have led the public to distrust death-
rate reporting, but we were not stupid in Oxford. Having
won that battle, we knew that the system would search
for some other reason to close us down.

Other centres soon came under attack. The press simply
failed to grasp that in any statistical ranking 50 per cent
of surgeons or hospitals would sit below average. When
the overall children's survival rate in Glasgow was
reported as 95.9 per cent against the UK average of 96.7
per cent there was a public outcry. The Scottish press
complained, 'Death rates for paediatric heart operations
in Glasgow were significantly higher than in the rest of
the UK.' A whole 0.8 per cent higher! The chairperson of
the Scottish Patients Association moaned, 'This is totally
unacceptable and I am very concerned! The hospital may
be happy with its figures but I am not!' Local television
gave coverage to the attack, which eroded confidence in a
thoroughly reputable centre.

Then came Safe and Sustainable, a full-blown political
initiative aimed at closing almost half of the children's
heart surgery centres in England, including the Royal
Brompton Hospital. A committee of strategically selected
political activists was assembled, who then set about deni-
grating centres other than their own. Safe and Sustainable
decreed that surviving centres should have at least four
children's heart surgeons. Few units had that many and,
despite claims to the contrary, there was no evidence that
bigger was better. Indeed, most units in the United States
were smaller than Oxford. Predictably, this prompted a

recruitment drive to bring in children's heart surgeons from overseas in a quest for survival. Worse still, my only paediatric colleague had returned to his homeland Sri Lanka to establish a unit there, leaving me to work single-handed again.

By now Oxford was ambivalent about whether it could afford to keep the programme should it prove to be more expensive in the future. Yet the poor parents and the region that we served were desperate to keep us. Under pressure from the public, the John Radcliffe Hospital looked for two new paediatric cardiac surgeons. Despite the prestige of Oxford, the only suitable applicants came from overseas. One excellent candidate was an established surgeon from Norway who had trained with me for two years, but he had to withdraw because the move would halve his salary. The second came on a temporary basis, having worked successfully as a consultant independently in a top Australian hospital. By the time he arrived I had been working single-handed for more than two years with no downtime whatsoever. It was approaching the festive season and I was actually told by the management to take the leave owed to me or lose it altogether. With another fully trained surgeon in-house and my family to look after, it seemed a reasonable thing to do.

In my absence over Christmas there was an unprece-dented run of complex emergency cases – and some of them died. Hearing about this, I decided that the unit should stop operating until the circumstances of the deaths were understood and the new surgeon exonerated from blame. But I already knew that this was the chance

the authorities were waiting for. They would use it to reinforce their case that smaller centres should close. Yet
another inquiry was what they needed to kick-start the
Safe and Sustainable process. The committee were keen to
rake through my results too, undoubtedly in an attempt
to discredit the whole unit as in Bristol. But they could
not fault my results, nor did they criticise the other
surgeon; he subsequently left Oxford, as we knew he had
planned to do, becoming a successful surgeon elsewhere.
Nevertheless, the frustrated authorities decided that we
should not resume operating until we had recruited more
surgeons. Perfectly reasonable, but we all knew that this
would be impossible as there were none to recruit. Why
would anyone want to be a children's heart surgeon in
this environment?

When we closed to babies and children I was finally
relieved of the continuous on-call commitment and my
self-imposed embargo on alcohol consumption. Certainly,
I would miss operating on children, but I simply threw the
switch and walked away from it all, liberated from this
huge responsibility. But at what price? Perhaps the best
facilities for academic paediatric surgery in England were
now redundant, and all the expertise I had developed with
Wilson to perform combined catheter interventions with
less invasive cardiac surgery was wasted, as were our
facilities in the charitably funded children's hospital.
Moreover, the regional premature baby unit no longer
possessed a surgeon to clip the ductus arteriosus when it
failed to close spontaneously, and newborn infants from
our whole region had to travel all the way to Southampton

or London for a fifteen-minute procedure that I would normally perform in their cot.

The parents were devastated, especially those whose kids had undergone a palliative procedure and were waiting for me to perform a second corrective operation. They trusted the Oxford team, but now had to travel many miles to surgeons they had never previously met. All our protests went unheeded. Without surgical backup, Neil Wilson could not perform his sophisticated techniques in the catheter laboratory, so he left to head up a unit in Denver, Colorado. Then with their own units under wider threat of closure, other respected surgeons decided to emigrate to America or return to their own countries. Other hospitals challenged with closure fought the process. When allegations of 'inappropriate process' and misinformation were used against Safe and Sustainable in court – which we had rechristened 'Dodgy and Distainable' – the whole process was discredited and thrown out. As a result, the other threatened centres remain open years later.

After our paediatric service was closed down, other children were not as lucky as Oliver. By then I was involved with a number of different and exciting projects, such as the artificial hearts and cardiac stem cells, but I missed the immense satisfaction that comes from saving a child. Who else gets messages like this last line from Nicky's letter?

I know how lucky we were as a family to have had
you in our lives for that brief moment of time. Every
day for us, every family get together, every Christmas
or special occasion is that much happier for what you
did. Thank you. Thank you. Thank you!

What better legacy than that?

11

misery

ONE REVIEWER OF *Fragile Lives* in a national newspaper questioned my overt 'lack of self-doubt'. This delicate soul had clearly become accustomed to medical writers who peddle introspection and vulnerability as their theme. But believe me, self-doubt is no more a desirable attribute in an experienced heart surgeon than in a sniper in Afghanistan. We both have a job to do. When I perform well, the patient benefits; if I don't get it right, they die. If the sniper hits his target, the terrorist dies; should he fail to blow their brains out, the terrorist will kill his colleagues. Simple. How does introspection and self-doubt help with that?

I know, however, where this touchy-feely stuff is coming from. The General Medical Council revalidation process requires us to be inward-looking and reflect on our practice, and the legally binding Duty of Candour orders us to tell the truth to our patients or in my case their bereaved relatives. So let me finally share some self-doubt with you and explain why I eventually had to walk away from it all.

The duty hospital administrator tracked me down and bluntly insisted that I admit a patient to our ward because he was about to breach the four-hour waiting-time target in the accident department. This would snatch our last bed from a deteriorating heart failure patient who was scheduled for both aortic and mitral valve replacements the following day. But the manager was only doing his job, so I politely informed him that I'd come down in five minutes and if he cared to push the waiting patient out into the hospital corridor he could dutifully tick his box.

Now I needed to know more about the gentleman being forcibly admitted into my care. He was a fit young builder who had slipped down a staircase on the job, bounced on his right lower chest and experienced local-ised severe pain, which, with a couple of cracked ribs, was hardly surprising. His concerned work mates called 999 and a massively expensive helicopter with a doctor on board was dispatched to the building site. First, let me pre-empt the ongoing discussion by stating that the pre-hospital emergency services save many thousands of lives. But on this occasion there was another passenger along for the ride – a cameraman. A television production company was making a documentary about the magnifi-cent men in their flying machines, so there had to be a bit of drama in the form of an intravenous drip and chest drain inserted amid the dust and rubble of the building site.

You will appreciate by now that a chest drain is used to remove blood or air from that potential space around the lung known as the pleural cavity. I say 'potential' because there is no space between the lung and chest wall unless air has leaked or bleeding has occurred from traumatised arteries in the chest wall. I have no doubt that the doctor had the best of intentions and followed the guidelines for helicopter retrieval at the time, but we normally only insert a chest drain following a chest X-ray so we know what we are treating and precisely where to position it. I have seen a number of these tubes pushed directly into the heart, with fatal consequences.

To insert the drain the doctor injected local anaesthetic between the ribs, then made a stab wound through the chest wall with a scalpel. The plastic tube was pushed into the builder's chest to evacuate whatever was compromising his breathing, despite the fact that he was neither shocked nor short of breath. He was just bloody sore and doubtless could have walked to the hospital for a chest X-ray. But the man was now certainly bewildered, because the drain made the pain even worse. Nor did he need intravenous fluids – he was anxious and his blood pressure was already elevated. Nevertheless, all of this would doubtless make great television and help raise funds for the air ambulance.

When the patient eventually reached the hospital, a chest X-ray showed the chest drain to be deeply embedded within the substance of the right lung. Why? Because there had never been anywhere to put it – no space created by blood or air. Fibrous adhesions from a previous chest infection had obliterated the right pleural cavity, and he now had a penetrating stab wound of the lung. He did have two undisplaced cracked ribs, but I have played rugby with similar after a few millilitres of local anaesthetic.

Irritated by the prospect of cancelling my own patient, I simply told the doctors in this regional trauma centre to pull out the drain, place a dressing over the wound and send him home with a packet of paracetamol. This is what they do in Cape Town and Johannesburg, otherwise their hospital beds would be overflowing with stab wounds. But none of these doctors had the confidence to do that as they were all filled with self-doubt and introspection. What if something went wrong? Everyone would be sued. So I had to take him to the cardiothoracic ward and do it myself, while the poor heart failure patient was sent home, leaving me with a costly gap on my operating list the following day.

But what about the builder? When his wife asked me whether he needed the chest drain, I had to tell her that he didn't. Duty of Candour. The reason he was sitting in the ward was a stab wound that bore absolutely no relation to his bruised ribs. He would have been safer coming to hospital by car, if at all. This was just what published Washington Trauma Center studies showed for penetrating injuries. Pre-hospital care can be over-invasive; swoop, scoop and run saves lives. Needless to say, the television programme did not broadcast the sequence – but they should have done. Unless these issues are openly discussed, no one will learn from them. As a young man I wrote and edited two textbooks on chest trauma, and fought hard to have helicopter retrieval introduced to Britain after my experiences in America. But helicopters are only useful for life-threatening problems that need rapid transport over long distances. They are only as effective as those who direct them.

Contrast this aerial drama with the mundane reality of our routine out-of-hours medical services. To be fair, the good old NHS had been good to my parents. My father had a potentially fatal heart attack aborted by a cardiologist friend, who quickly and decisively placed a stent in his occluded coronary artery. My dear mother was operated on very successfully for three separate cancers by colleagues who were determined to do their best for her. And indeed for me. But that was while I still worked in the NHS and had some influence over their care.

March 2016, a Saturday morning. My mother's two carers roused her, then transferred her from her bed to a chair. One of the carers was recovering from the winter flu bug, but there was no slack in the system. She had to work. At ninety-two, with dementia and severe Parkinson's disease, my mother's life had been restricted to that one room for five years, although she was content enough in her own world. Father had been deaf since working on heavy bombers in the Second World War and was now virtually blind from macular degeneration. But at ninety-four he remained my mother's constant companion and they were happy together in their own home. Depending upon when I could extricate myself from the hospital, either my wife Sarah or I would feed them every evening.

That morning during the intensive care round, Sarah called me on the mobile. My mother was uncomfortable, with rattling lungs and a temperature, and Dad thought we would wish to know. I realised that this would spell the end for her, so I picked up Sarah and we drove to the house to get some grasp on the situation. Mum was slumped in her reclining chair, clearly agitated and breathing heavily. Her pulse rate was 120 beats per minute and her lips had that slate blue tinge that I recognised only too well. Although her hands were cold and clammy, her forehead was hot, and from my father's expression I realised that he knew the score. We all wanted her to be comfortable and relieved of distress. I knew how to achieve that. I was there when my grandfather's kindly GP came to the house when he was dying from heart failure. Morphine helped him on his way. As a junior doctor in the 1970s I did the same for many desperate patients. It is what compassionate doctors do. 'End of life' care, and common decency.

I decided to call my mother's geriatrician Dr Singh, who asked whether we wanted to bring her into the hospital. I explained that I thought she was going to die and that we didn't want her to be dragged off by strangers in an ambulance to the corridors of a crowded A&E department. We wanted her to slip away peacefully in her own home, surrounded by family and with the dignity she deserved. I didn't even want to move her back to the bed. Dr Singh's wise advice was not to make any intervention myself. For obvious legal reasons we should call a GP, just as my dear mother had done for her father sixty years ago. So I set about trying to find medical help on a Saturday.

Thanks to the Labour government, NHS GPs were given a pay rise in 2003 for abrogating all responsibility for patients outside daytime working hours and at weekends. The much-cherished family doctor was terminated for reasons of financial and political expediency. Out-of-practice hours is now a Russian roulette system in which the sick either take themselves to hospital or call a help line known as NHS 111, a deeply frustrating system introduced by the Conservative government that shifted decision-making from doctors to lay call handlers. The public were told: 'If you need immediate emergency help, call 999. For all other urgent healthcare needs, there is 111. If you need to see a GP urgently, the service will make sure this happens. If you need to see a nurse or need an urgent home visit out of working hours, NHS 111 will organise it.' How reassuring was that!

At midday, this professor of surgery dials 111 and a dialogue of incomprehensible stupidity begins. The lay call handler reads out her lines – 'Do you need an ambulance?' I reply with clarity that my beloved mother is dying and I would like her to be relieved of the breathlessness and distress that she is currently suffering. She needs the kind attention of a GP in her own home. I then receive a barrage of wholly inappropriate questions about whether she is still breathing or bleeding and lots of other crap, none of which bears any relevance whatsoever to the reality of the situation. I become more assertive. I am a doctor. I know what the patient needs. I do not need someone who may have worked in Sainsbury's last week to reconsider that decision. The call handler is now confused, unable to depart from protocol. She will get her supervisor to call me back. This reminded me starkly of my adventures in China in 1978, but even the so-called 'barefoot doctors' were better!

I sat holding my mother's hand, intermittently checking her faltering pulse. Short of oxygen, her strong heart had slipped into rapid atrial fibrillation. The telephone was still clutched in my other fist. When it rang, my mother stirred, coughed, then dribbled blood-stained fluid from her nose. The same ridiculous process began once again, with the same inane questions. I made it clear that I did not want an ambulance to bring my mother to hospital. The conversation was going nowhere. Our situation was deteriorating and I sensed that there was no help to be had.

'I will get our medical officer [the one sitting in the call centre directing traffic] to call you on this number,' the frustrated woman eventually told me.

After further delay the doctor called, and I left him in no doubt about the nature of the situation and what I believed should happen. Even he took some persuading, but he agreed to send the single GP covering the whole region. I just wanted my poor mother to have some morphine. In the meantime, Sarah the nurse made her as comfortable as possible, moistening her lips and cooling her brow with a cold flannel.

Then her breathing changed perceptibly from its regular, laboured, heaving pattern to an intermittent, irregular gasping that doctors call Cheyne–Stokes respiration. Now I knew she didn't need the doctor anymore. Divine help had arrived. Her pulse was thready and slowing. Her eyes rolled, then remained shut. Her breaths became more intermittent, eventually fading away altogether. I looked at my distraught father and stated the obvious. She's gone.

I don't need to explain how it feels when your mother dies, but death for her came as a great relief. Relief that – in 2016 – she couldn't access from the medical profession. I guess I wanted that doctor to arrive more than my mother did. I needed to tell myself that I had done everything possible to help her when the time came. Yet the system I'd toiled in without a single day of sick leave in more than forty years had finally let me down when my family needed it. I became increasingly bitter about that.

A very sympathetic lady GP arrived at 4.30 pm, ten minutes after the passing, four and a half hours after I'd sought help. She was profoundly embarrassed and described the system as in chaos, which meant she couldn't reach us any sooner. It was fitting testament to a broken NHS. It made no difference that our family was full of doctors. No one was there to help. My mother died peacefully at home, surrounded by her family. Had she lived in a nursing home, an ambulance would have shipped her off to the accident department to die on a trolley in a busy hospital corridor.

June 2016. I was in the hospital late in the afternoon when my lawyer daughter Gemma called me in a state of anxiety. Unusual for her, but my eighteen-month-old granddaughter was vomiting repeatedly, couldn't keep anything down and was becoming lethargic and floppy. When my daughter rang the GP's surgery, she was told that there were no more appointments that day so she should find a pharmacy for advice, which is what is recommended by NHS England. Having done just this, the young lady pharmacist was hesitant to offer any opinion on a dehydrated child and suggested the 111 route. Halfway through these discussions my daughter decided that she had no confidence whatsoever in what she was hearing, so she called me in Oxford to ask my advice.

As a paediatric surgeon, certain words triggered alarm bells for me. 'Lethargic and floppy' in a baby often spells low blood sugar and immediate danger, so I told Gemma to go directly to the children's emergency department at Addenbrooke's Hospital in Cambridge, and I called the unit myself, hoping that they would be seen on arrival.

I let Gemma know that she was not alone in abandoning the prescribed process, as a great number of intelligent patients abandon 111 calls. The chair of the British Medical Associations General Practitioners Committee referred to 111 as a 'disaster zone' because of the number of calls that were inappropriately triaged. It was a relief that the kindly sister in charge at Addenbrooke's was happy to take my call. I then set off on the dreaded M40, M25, A1 journey to my old hospital in the middle of rush hour. Few things can be more stressful than a distant medical emergency in your own family. When I arrived, the little bundle was being rehydrated with glucose through a drip in her arm. Everyone felt safe by now –

great hospital, great doctors and nurses. It was getting her there that was the problem.

Within twelve months I received another urgent call from Essex. Returning from the school run, Gemma witnessed a little old lady stumble into the main road and fall heavily on her face. Gemma stopped her car in a position to shield the woman from oncoming traffic. Covered in abrasions and bruises, the victim was in great pain and appeared to have a fractured collar bone, so Gemma stayed at the roadside and asked another passer-by to fetch the lady's elderly husband, who brought a chair and sat beside his prostrate spouse. It was a bizarre tableau, but no one felt confident enough to shift the poor, immobile woman. The obvious course of action was to call for an ambulance, which is precisely what Gemma did.

Once again my lawyer daughter was faced by the rote of triage questions: 'Is she breathing, is she bleeding, can you see the baby's head? Sorry, wrong questionnaire.' I jest, obviously, but after a frustrating and mostly pointless set of questions she was told that an ambulance would be on its way, but it could take up to four hours. As it turned out it wasn't as bad as that; it was three hours and forty minutes. As my daughter sat comforting the pair, someone else directed the traffic around this human obstruction.

A passing fire engine stopped to enquire about the incident. What they said was along the lines of 'Don't blame the ambulance service. Their vehicles are queuing outside the hospital waiting to unload. The accident department is full because they can't send any patients to the wards.

The wards are full because they can't discharge their patients into the community. A quarter of the beds are occupied by patients who don't need to be there, but there is nowhere else to look after them.'

My daughter thanked them for their reassuring insight and they moved on. The elderly lady was hypothermic when she eventually reached Addenbrooke's, just ten miles away.

What do Albert Einstein and our treasured NHS have in common? Answer: they were brilliant for their time, but when they reached seventy they both died from something eminently treatable. In Einstein's case, it was an aortic aneurysm for which he persistently refused surgery, a common obstinacy and resistance to change that is difficult to understand. For the NHS, it's the 'free for all at the point of delivery' principle that is impossible to sustain because the population is aging and only a proportion of us pay taxes to pay for it. And free healthcare has long been a tourist industry.

The NHS of 2018 is unrecognisable from how it used to be in 1948, when it was established. Modern medicine relies on thousands of drugs and increasingly complex technology, both of which have become vastly more expensive with time. My own specialty has changed immeasurably since I came to Oxford in 1986. Much of the surgery we did for coronary artery disease has been superseded by coronary stenting under local anaesthetic, often on a day-case basis. When performed during a heart attack, this technique restores blood flow to the dying muscle and if done in time can salvage a significant amount of it. Some of those saved do go on to suffer heart failure, but they might soon receive an injection of stem cells down that catheter too. Even though the results are marginally better with coronary bypass surgery, who would honestly prefer a foot-long incision up the sternum and another in the leg or arm to harvest the graft conduits?

Even prosthetic heart valves can now be inserted by a cardiologist. They are rolled on to the end of a catheter, then unfurled forcibly within the diseased valve, an approach that is already routine in older age groups in some European countries. Less invasive techniques are being developed for the mitral valve, but in those for whom conventional mitral valve surgery remains preferable, this can now be undertaken through a small incision in the right chest wall supported by robotics or enabling technology.

Most abdominal aortic aneurysms, such as the one that killed Einstein, no longer need open surgery through a large abdominal incision. An endovascular stent graft, usually deployed on a catheter from the groin under detailed X-ray screening, excludes the swollen part of the aorta from within. The same innovative techniques are suitable for many aneurysms in the chest, and they hugely reduced the volume of my aortic surgery practice. Instead of ten days in hospital following major open surgery with cooling and circulatory arrest, the patient can often go home by the end of the day. In children with congenital heart disease, narrowed vessels can be dilated then stented open, while abnormal vessels and holes in the heart can be closed using catheter-based technology. My talented colleague Neil Wilson was the UK's leading light in this respect, but he had to emigrate to carry on.

And finally back to heart failure, the only fatal disease with a worse prognosis than cancer. Those suffering from it experience breathlessness on the slightest exertion, constant physical exhaustion, an inability to lie flat, a distended abdomen and legs, then complete dependence upon others. I am really proud of my efforts to develop an alternative to heart transplantation, but although I first implanted a permanent rotary blood pump in 2000, in 2018 these pumps have yet to be made available for the thousands of terminally ill patients under sixty-five years old in the UK who are not eligible for one of the handful of donor hearts. Even with this brutally ageist approach, less than 1 per cent of those who might benefit from a transplant ever receive a donor organ. How would you feel if your son or daughter were dying from heart failure? If the system cannot provide lifesaving technology, change the system.

I last vented my frustration on these issues at a conference at the Texas Heart Institute in September 2017. Although the meeting was called 'Advances in Cardiovascular Medicine', the convenors also wanted me to reflect on the seventy-year anniversary of socialised medicine. I declined to do that, as I had no desire to run down the NHS. But the Americans are not stupid – they are watching us carefully. When I witnessed practical demonstrations of their state-of-the-art technology I found myself reminded of another trip. I was in India, trying to reach the far side of a lake in Udaipur on a bakingly hot Rajasthan afternoon, but my taxi was held up by the untouchable sacred cows languishing in the road. On the horizon my destination shimmered into view, the opulent Lake Palace Hotel. The NHS is just such a sacred cow, and being in Houston again felt like looking across the waters of the lake in wonder at the opulence. How did we allow our beloved NHS to reach this situation?

In the 1990s my colleagues in Oxford and I each performed between 500 to 600 heart operations a year. We were a finely honed production line of cardiac surgery, with a great team and excellent results, and surgeons came from all across the world to observe what we had achieved. But it became politically incorrect to work that hard in the NHS and every opportunity was taken to criticise us. We were told we should be spending more time on surgical training, attending outreach clinics in far-flung general hospitals or participating in management meetings. Anything, in fact, apart from doing what we had been trained to do – something that others couldn't do – which was operate on sick hearts. Political correctness and the system eventually won out. Now the six cardiac surgeons at my hospital each perform around 150 operations per year, fewer than 1,000 cases a year between all of them.

2 January 2018. As the seventieth anniversary of the NHS kicked off, the newspaper headlines repeated the same old stories: '14 ambulances queuing to discharge patients outside one hospital yesterday'; 'Bed-blocked hospitals issue plea to relatives to take patients home';

'36-hour trolley wait for dementia patient'; 'Pensioner dies from heart attack after 4-hour wait for an ambulance'; '24 NHS trusts on black alert since New Year'; '55,000 planned operations cancelled this month'.

And so it went on. A prominent politician described going off to Europe for brain cancer treatment that was unavailable on the NHS. A baby with a heart tumour must go to the Massachusetts General Hospital for surgery because no one can do it in the UK. So is our NHS the envy of the world? I really don't think so. It has just become more financially adept, saving money before saving lives.

On 11 January, sixty-eight senior consultants representing half of the A&E departments in the country wrote to the prime minister, saying that 'patients are dying in hospital corridors amid intolerable NHS conditions.' This was no exaggeration – a toxic combination of rising demand, jam-packed hospitals and wholly inadequate social care had created a tidal wave that swamped our understaffed and under-resourced emergency departments. But better to wait for hours to be seen than not be seen at all. My friend Chris Bulstrode was Professor of Orthopaedics at Oxford University before he retired early to retrain as an emergency medicine doctor. He provided an interesting perspective on the role of A&E following the demise of family GPs:

It should really be called the department for patients no one else wants. If the police can't cope with a mentally ill person or the family can't cope with an elderly relative or a GP can't solicit an urgent outpatient appointment, they just send them to the emergency department. I fear that if we don't do something radical soon the system will collapse and bring the whole NHS down with it.

Many of us share his sentiments and fear that the politicians have misjudged the mood. The situation in early 2018 was chaotic and impossible to comprehend, unless you witnessed it for yourself. The prime minister responded by declaring that 'the NHS is better funded than ever before' and 'better prepared for this winter than ever before'. All we hear from politicians is the same fantasy and deceit. Apparently, the suspension of elective operations that rendered many thousands of staff and their facilities idle was all part of the seasonal 'masterplan'. For the past ten years, these same senior figures presided over thousands of hospital bed closures, the disintegration of mental health and social services, and the damaging alienation of the medical and nursing professions. What's more, the perpetual overseas recruitment drive that aims to poach trained staff from the developing world is a disgrace in itself.

Those who ask whether I would follow the same career path again usually appreciate the immeasurable time and effort put into the role and the impact this has had on any semblance of family life. When I trained, then during the early years of my consultant career, we worked in a more supportive environment alongside teams brimming with enthusiasm. Although I was repeatedly chastised for going off piste to save lives, it was usually with the wag of a finger and a grin, followed by the profound gratitude of a grateful family. These days it would be instant 'gardening leave' followed by a lawsuit – assuming that the patient hadn't brought one first. So who takes these chances now?

Before answering, I sometimes relate the story of what happened to the surgical pioneer Charles Bailey after he'd achieved that first successful mitral valvotomy in the United States. For a while he was a hero, but before long he was subject to three lawsuits in Philadelphia. These outraged him, and, disillusioned by the increasingly litigious environment, he simply quit surgery, retrained in law and joined the lucrative medico-legal business himself.

Clearly, some cases of clinical negligence are justified. But I refer to it as a business because that is exactly what it is. Anyone who feels aggrieved about any aspect of their care can now formulate a complaint and mount a 'no win, no fee' fishing expedition at the NHS's expense. So-called medical experts line up to siphon off any extra cash they can make. The lawyers get paid a fortune and sometimes the patient emerges intact. Often they don't. They then spend the rest of their lives feeling aggrieved and depressed about something that they should simply have discussed with their surgeon. But from our perspective, the NHS, with its focus on death and misery, has encouraged doctor-bashing instead of putting a stop to it.

So returning to the question as to whether I would train in cardiac surgery in the current era, sadly the answer is no. I would do a 'Charles Bailey' and study law just as my daughter did. But would I do it again with my old expansive practice in a well-equipped centre, within an environment where safety mattered more than money? You bet. I gained inordinate pleasure from helping frightened patients and their families through the most uncertain episode of their lives, as well as enormous satisfaction simply from the technical aspects of repairing a failing heart and watching a person walk out of the hospital into a new life. Fragile lives made better. But we shouldn't have to jump through hoops for that privilege. There are plenty of other countries where cardiac surgeons are still highly valued.

I was now sixty-eight and waiting for surgery on a deformed right hand where the nurses had smacked heavy metal instruments into my palm. Could I face any more GMC revalidation questionnaires, any more mind-numbing 'statutory and mandatory' training? Absolutely not. After almost forty years in heart surgery, I knew it was time to move on. So I simply walked out of the hospital one Friday evening and never went back. No Festschrift, no card, no present. But also no regrets – and a huge sense of relief. I had new plans and ambitions. I was already a professor at the University of Swansea, where our bioengineers were working on the new miniature artificial heart, and now a professor at the Royal Brompton, where we were about to undertake a clinical trial with those magic genetically engineered stem cells that removed scar from the left ventricle after a heart attack.

12

fear

THAT CALAMITY ON THE CORNISH rugby pitch might have shaped my destiny, but it also left me prone to intrusive flashbacks. These spontaneous visual spectacles would invade my thoughts seemingly at random, without any conscious attempt to draw them from memory. It took me a while to realise that there were triggers for the hallucinations. The odour of a particular disinfectant might take me back to the Harlem trauma room where I was stabbed by a drug addict or to the rural Chinese hospital after the Cultural Revolution where I had joined the barefoot doctors to save children dying from dysentery. Just a whiff of burned toast could retrieve gruesome images of the sternal saw tearing through bone into the right ventricle. In the midst of a flashback I was unable to distinguish fantasy from reality. So I always kept them to myself, and once they passed they really didn't trouble me, just like the prodromal flashing lights of my migraine headaches.

My training in the United States coincided with the finale of the Vietnam War. In Alabama I met several veterans who suffered repeated flashbacks of death and destruction that caused them anxiety and insomnia, ultimately leading to depression or crime. It was a problem also seen in rape victims and Holocaust survivors. In 1980 the American Psychiatric Association named this syndrome 'post-traumatic stress disorder'. Since then, sophisticated brain-imaging techniques have shown that deeply traumatic events interfere with the normal mechanisms by which memories are stored. Moreover, my Phineas Gage phenomenon undoubtedly had an interface with these neural pathways.

The hippocampus is the brain's depository for day-to day-memories that are amenable to conscious recall. In turn, the pea-sized amygdala selects out emotional memories of the fear-generating type. Some consider that the amygdala evolved specifically to promote survival through encoding danger. Thus, an individual will rapidly recognise a significant threat if encountered again. Preferentially, the two centres cooperate to encode all experience in long-term memory, but an adrenaline-fuelled fight-or-flight reaction will overstimulate the amygdala while supressing the hippocampus. The creation of cohesive memory is then deprioritised to favour reflex response to danger.

In threatening circumstances that recall a traumatic event, the amygdala spews the memory back into the conscious brain in an unregulated manner. This is why flashbacks automatically activate the sympathetic nervous system, causing rapid heart rate, sweating and heavy breathing in addition to the fear. Because the hippocampus wasn't keyed in properly to the original trauma, the contextual element of the memory wasn't stored, so no feedback exists to convince the amygdala that the danger no longer exists. Straightforward neuropsychology – or is it?

It's easy to understand how my own head trauma that disrupted my ability to register fear, was linked to my propensity for flashbacks and, wholly positively, gave me the courage to be different. I was never concerned about departing from protocol or trying something new, nor was I perturbed by risk. As I've said before, it wasn't me on the operating table. In retrospect, however, I would certainly have avoided some of the inordinately difficult cases had I not been disinhibited at the time. It was the same in my personal life. I consistently drove stupidly fast and on occasion performed reckless deeds to help others in dire circumstances. Sometimes the recklessness was construed as bravery, but it was nothing of the sort – I simply didn't appreciate danger as others might.

Over the years my psyche gradually reverted to normal, whatever normal is. As apprehension and common sense intervened, my professional life became progressively more uncomfortable, not just psychologically but physically too. In recent years my testosterone-fuelled existence predisposed me to prostatic hypertrophy and miserable urinary symptoms – urgency, poor stream, dribbling, the inability to stand through a whole operation and the need to get up several times each night. Eventually I developed such a fear of urinary retention, fuelled by my own grim endeavours to relieve that problem for others while a urology registrar in Cambridge, that I always travelled abroad with a urinary catheter in my hand luggage.

Eventually aging mind and disintegrating body came together when I experienced anxiety and desperation during a difficult operation, and it was all I could do not to piss my pants. I was attempting to repair a huge aortic arch aneurysm that involved the main blood vessels to the brain, an operation that other surgeons were keen to avoid. Worse still, the patient was a well-known professor at the university whom I knew quite well. Whether I liked it or not, this personal bond carried a particular responsibility. It was another case, involving stopping the circulation, draining out his blood and replacing the aortic arch against the clock. What's more, this was not a cerebral cortex I could risk damaging …

Forty minutes is the safe duration for circulatory arrest, because at 18°C the brain's metabolism and oxygen consumption is lowered to 20 per cent of normal. Any longer without blood flow risks brain damage, which worsens by the minute. Unusually I had no reservations whatsoever about that, as I was a plumber who specialised in large aneurysms and had always regarded surgery as an emotionless, technical exercise, comparable to lifting the bonnet of an automobile and repairing the engine. Done skilfully in a reasonable time frame, the patient will survive and prosper. Take too long or bugger it up, then that great hospital in the sky beckons.

I had the aorta wide open and was staring up the two horribly diseased carotid arteries that passed directly into the professor's distinguished cranium. Both resembled water pipes clogged with limescale. Atheromatous plaques throughout the aortic arch disintegrated on touch, oozing liquid fat like pus. And I was meant to sew a pristine polyester graft to this stuff, then re-implant those crappy carotid vessels, when the slightest speck of debris that detached itself and ended up in the brain could cause a devastating stroke. As I started sewing the diseased arteries they began to disintegrate. I remember thinking, 'Bugger, will I get this together in time? Yes, I'll get it sorted, but then again it's possible I won't. Shit. Maybe today, just when the whole of Oxford is watching, it will all fall to bits.' And, of course, it did.

I completed the three suture lines, proximal and distal on the aorta, together with separate implantation of the head vessels. Then I asked the perfusionist to pump a few hundred millilitres of blood from his machine to displace air from the graft, while I hummed 'Air in the brain, life down the drain.' At low pressure the repair seemed watertight, but when we reached full flow the distal anastomosis gave way in the back of the chest and blood hosed out into the suckers.

'So who's the sucker now?' I thought. At that point it seemed like my own blood had drained from me. Streams of sweat ran down my back and I felt cold, as if my adrenal glands had been wiped out. It had already taken me thirty-five minutes of circulatory arrest to replace the whole arch, so I was really up against it. With no alternative other than to stop the pump, drain the blood again and re-sew the dehisced suture line, it would be a struggle to keep his brain alive.

This time I used a larger needle with deeper bites and a thick strip of Teflon felt to buttress tissues that possessed all the tensile strength of Stilton. The process took another fifteen minutes of intense concentration, interspersed with bad-tempered exchanges with fearful assistants who were only trying to be helpful, 'trying' being the operative word.

Because the circulatory arrest time was beyond the edge of tolerance, the de-airing was perfunctory and he was quickly put back onto cardiopulmonary bypass with a view to rewarming. For another couple of minutes the stitch lines stayed dry, his brain gratefully extracted some oxygen and my mood lifted. Then blood suddenly began to squirt like a fountain from where the head arteries had been re-implanted into the graft. I tried to insert a few extra buttressed stitches while still on the bypass machine, but the needle tore the tissues again and made things worse. Just when 'Mr Unflappable' needed an uncomplicated home run, I began to despair.

The spectre of this famous Oxford scientist reduced to a vegetable or terminated by his overconfident surgeon loomed large, and I could anticipate how it would be described in the obituary columns. I thought about what Sarah taught her nurses to do when they were emotionally extended in the accident department – 'Take slow, deep breaths.' Deep breathing stimulates the parasympathetic nervous system, the stress-mitigating opposite of the adrenaline-fuelled panic reaction and the basis for mindfulness. She would say, 'Feel your body. Jettison the turmoil your empathy leaves you vulnerable to. Feel your feet on the floor and wiggle your toes. That helps you out of your patient's shoes and back into your own.' A wise woman.

I succeeded in entering that mental tunnel, forcing everything out of my mind but the sheer practicality of sewing rapidly, as if I were stitching a cardboard toilet roll or a tear in my pants. The anaesthetist was agitated, the perfusionist was counting the minutes out loud and the assistants had all turned to jelly. But between us we succeeded in keeping it together and completing the operation. The man's entire nervous system had experienced sixty-five minutes without blood flow and I fully expected a dismal outcome. Beyond the cerebral hypoxia, the risk of stroke from air embolism or detached chunks of atheroma was huge. What was I going I tell his poor wife? That was a conversation to avoid until the next case was finished. I had suffered enough emotional contagion for one day, whatever that means.

I did what I was now compelled to do after separating from the bypass machine – I took a step backwards, tossed away my bloodied gloves and nodded to the registrar to close up. Pretending to head for coffee, I made directly for the surgeons' changing room to discharge my aching irritable bladder. Then horror of horrors. Out dribbled bright red wine, followed by frank blood. 'Oh shit!' was my immediate thought. 'I've got the Big C.' I suspected that a stress-related surge in blood pressure had caused either a prostate or bladder tumour to bleed. With an aortic valve replacement still to do, my volatile mood descended into my boots – sheer panic would be a more realistic description.

Type A personalities seek rapid resolution to any worrying issue. Tedious symptoms from benign prostatic enlargement were one thing; bleeding cancer was quite another, ratcheting my anxiety up a considerable number of gears. If feasible, I needed to dispel this worry before the next case. Most people would have to wait a week to see their GP, then months for an appointment with a urologist. I simply dialled the mobile number of my close colleague David Cranston. We operated together on kidney tumours that had spread up the veins and into the heart. I would put the patient on the bypass machine, then drain the circulation just as I had done that morning. David would dissect out and remove the cancer from the inferior vena cava, then I would repair it with a tube or patch. Operating on large blood vessels is simpler when they are empty. And for me, my next operation would be much more relaxed without blood dripping out of my penis. But what were the chances of finding David on this first frantic call?

He answered on the third ring tone.

'What are you doing right now, Dave?'

'An outpatient cystoscopy list.'

'Perfect,' I said, and I meant it, as cystoscopy is the examination of the prostate and bladder through a fibre optic telescope. 'Can you fit me in if I come straight across?'

The urology department is located in Oxford's Churchill Hospital, a short drive across town. I went out to the car park wearing theatre blues and in ten minutes pulled into the No Parking area at the Churchill main entrance. Just another five minutes and I was reclining on the examination couch with my legs in the air, my backside on display and a thick black pipe up my urethra. Uncomfortable, but ultimately satisfying. There was no sign of a bleeding tumour, just dilated veins on the inner surface of the prostate gland that had ruptured and clotted off. Once I'd been given the all clear, the removal of that pipe from my penis was one of life's great pleasures. I was back in my own operating theatre in less than ten minutes, with the next patient still awake in the anaesthetic room. Everyone thought that I had just popped out to my office.

Once it showed up, I found fear to be a miserably oppressive experience that I could well do without. Had every complex operation provoked these unpleasant responses I would have ditched the specialty much sooner, preferring to operate on bones or guts. Or better still, trained as a barrister and used penetrating words rather than sharp instruments. I wondered precisely what had triggered this emotional rollercoaster while operating on my professor friend. Was it just a rational response to the likelihood of losing a patient, a reaction that I had missed out on thus far? Did surgeons who lacked the benefit of my curiously rewired brain suffer regularly in such circumstances? Or was consideration for my friend something to do with it? Empathy is something I experience perpetually for my own close family, but it would be fucking madness and wholly counterproductive for surgeons to feel the same for every sick patient.

Clearly, the more empathetic we are, the more likely we are to be miserable ourselves. Sarah worked at the sharp end and referred to it as 'compassion fatigue'. It is the fast track to burnout – and I knew several surgeons with burnout. They ended up apathetic, depersonalised, exhausted and withdrawn, ground down by their working environment. I had always been resistant to all that, but today I saw how it could happen. I was on the verge of destroying my patient's brain when everyone was expecting me to cure him. But what was the panic really about? His potential demise or the straightforward risk to my own reputation?

I wasn't expecting the professor to regain consciousness that evening, but he did. I was still in my office when the night registrar bounced in to let me know. It cheered me up immensely, so I set off for intensive care to welcome him back to the land of the living. Waking up doesn't equate to intact intellect, but it's an important start. Might it be that the intermittent short bursts of brain reperfusion delivered sufficient oxygen to keep him safe, or did they just do enough to keep his brain stem alive? After all, he might still be a vegetable. These were my thoughts on the way there, but by the time I reached the bedside he was off the ventilator, tracheal tube out, and was talking to his wife. They registered my approach with unbridled, albeit undeserved, elation.

'Thank you, thank you, thank you. What a wonderful man,' was their greeting. But my steely eyes locked on to the blood pressure trace. The abrupt stimulus of waking had released a shedload of adrenaline, so the blood pressure was now far too high for a tenuous aorta. I could visualise the stitches cutting through like cheese wire, then unmitigated disaster as he deposited his whole blood volume into his chest. Sometimes I wished I had been a dermatologist. My gaze switched from the screen to the chest drains, as I politely asked the nurse what was being done to counter the lethal blood pressure.

I should have been greeting his grateful wife, lying to her about how well the operation had gone and taking the credit. But with a pressure of 180/110 mm Hg and possible exsanguination, I was verging on a hissy fit, a heart attack even. But if I said something offensive to those not looking after him I would be reported to the medical director for abusive behaviour. So again, I opted for mindfulness – 'Breathe deeply and feel calmer. Feel your body, then your feet on the floor.' Then I blasted the anaesthetic registrar for trying to kill my patient. Rather that than scream at the clueless agency nurse who remained oblivious as to what my issues were.

When I left, the professor's blood pressure spontaneously drifted down – the 'white-coat syndrome', not that I ever wore a white coat. When the patient sees a doctor coming, their blood pressure rises in response. Every time I went to the GP myself my blood pressure was too high, but when operating it used to be normal. I had been happy and relaxed plumbing hearts, at least until then.

I was sixty-eight when the contracture in my right hand curtailed my surgical career. The forty years of repeated slapping of metal instruments into my palm was the cause, and eventually I couldn't grasp them. I knew it would take months to recover from plastic surgery and return to work, but in all honesty I was bored with it all. I could no longer operate on patients with congenital heart disease and was unable to pursue my artificial heart and stem cell research in Oxford. I remained perfectly able to relieve suffering and extend lives, yet was actively prevented from doing so. While wondering about the morality of all that, I decided to move on. I could benefit more patients by dedicating time to these projects than by standing in an operating theatre for just a couple of days each week. But working with universities in other cities involved a fair amount of travel, and those wretched urological symptoms were catching up on me.

Surgeons never want surgery themselves. We know far too much about what can go wrong even in straightforward operations. During my urology training, prostatectomy carried two major complications – incontinence following relief of the obstruction, then impotence through damage to the nerves that regulate blood flow to the expandable parts I had valued for so long. This sobering memory from my years in training lingered with me over forty years later. On the other hand, how many prostate glands had I buggered up while trying to relieve the agony of urinary retention? For some, the alternative to the conventional but agonising catheter route was to stab a suprapubic tube directly into the bladder through the abdominal wall. Patients didn't object to that since it provided sweet relief from misery, which was all that mattered. So precarious was my situation that I still carried the catheter and anaesthetic gel everywhere I went. And for years I took a drug euphemistically named Flowmax. This enabled me to dribble marginally more effectively as I leaned precipitously forward against the bog wall.

Every year I took the prostate specific antigen blood test to exclude cancer. This remained persistently in the 'low risk' range, so I avoided going back to Professor Cranston. Then in 2017 two close cardiology friends who did not have urinary symptoms were diagnosed with prostate cancer. They could still piss with impunity, so what should I do when the antigen test was continuously rubbished as unreliable?

During the hot summer of 2018 I flew to Greece to review a series of patients whom, with my old trainees, I had injected with stem cells during coronary bypass surgery. Now a company doctor rather than a famous heart surgeon, I was obliged to travel in economy class. Predicting the inevitable, I purposefully dehydrated myself for the early morning flight. Nevertheless the urgency came on just as the drinks trolley blocked access to the lavatories at the back of the plane, leaving me with little choice but to seek relief forwards in the lightly subscribed business-class cabin. Sneaking through the blue curtain separating us plebs from the privileged few proved simple enough. But with my objective in clear sight I encountered a stroppy cabin services director helping herself to breakfast in the galley. Despite more than twenty years with frequent-flyer 'Gold Card' status, my path was blocked with grim determination.

'Economy passengers are not allowed in these toilets, sir,' she said. 'Your facilities are in the back of the aircraft.'

With that stern rebuke I leaked like a naughty school-boy and the urgency passed. You can image the social media coverage – 'Heart surgeon pisses his pants in panic'. Happy days. Eventually I made it to the queue at the rear of the aisle, resolving never to fly British Airways again. That resolution escalated to not flying at all until I'd had my miserable prostate bored out.

Any deliberation over the matter was now gone. Severe bladder outflow obstruction together with dehydration precipitated the crisis we call obstructive uropathy, an immediate threat to the kidneys. So after an uncomfortable return journey I called David Cranston that evening. Next day I met him in his clinic for another Dyno-Rod experience, followed by ultrasound scans of my prostate and bladder. These showed that my bladder simply didn't empty. I would waste minutes trying to piss but only pass one-third of the contents, like a rain barrel overflowing from time to time. Into the bargain it hurt, so I thought I had a urinary tract infection.

David was waiting for me to make my own mind up about surgery. In the interim I researched less radical alternatives. There is a new method of embolising the prostate's blood supply via a leg artery so that some of it dies and shrinks. Then there is the injection of pressurised steam to vaporise the obstructing tissue, but I visualised my penis blowing off like a factory whistle and didn't really fancy that. We drew the conclusion that it was not the time to piss around, in the colloquial sense. David's advice was to have the 'gold standard' transurethral resection, which is much safer than when I had a bash at it as a trainee. Back then it was done by peering up the narrow channel of a rigid metal instrument and burning away chunks of tissue with a hot wire. The residual gland would bleed profusely and fill the bladder with blood clots. Not surprisingly, I didn't much fancy that either in its earlier form.

Things were different now. My insides would be displayed with magnification on a television screen, the cutting could be carefully controlled, and the bleeding vessels seen and cauterised with a lower risk of complications: impotence 1 per cent, incontinence 1 per cent, I was told. For maximum enjoyment I could opt for a spinal anaesthetic and watch the televised proceedings myself. Not by any stretch of the imagination did I want to do that, nor have a needle probing around my spinal cord. Compared with my wife, then my daughter having their respective caesarean sections with regional anaesthesia, I was a complete coward.

Now down to the practicalities. Something had to be done soon to relieve the back pressure on my kidneys. I naively expected the surgery to be done in the NHS urology department, and as usual I wanted it to be done tomorrow. Then came sobering news. The best I could expect from the Churchill was an indwelling catheter to relieve the obstruction, then a place at the end of the waiting list. Why should that be after more than forty years of NHS service? Already there were 120 patients with benign prostatic hypertrophy on the waiting list, and many had

indwelling catheters already. They were not being operated on. Why? Because the surgeons were treading water
to keep up with cancer patients who had to be treated
within the government's prescribed time frame.
Regrettably I was not prepared to endure a year with a
pipe stuck up my penis and a bag of piss strapped to my
leg without guarantees at the end of that time, nor did I
want to progress to advanced kidney failure. So it was off
to the private hospital the following Saturday morning to
get it all over with.

It takes a conscious effort to switch from surgeon to
patient. Thanks to the miracle of modern anaesthesia and
surgical skill, the filleting and restoration of my claw hand
had been achieved as a day case. Now I was facing 'a few
days' in hospital, where I would have to adopt a passive
approach and do what I was told. As I agonised about
whom the anaesthetist should be, Sarah started fussing
around practical issues, such as 'I didn't own a dressing
gown or slippers.' The only pyjamas I possessed were a
gift from a kind patient with her own lingerie company
– bright blue pure silk, not quite the thing for a hospital
stay. So off Sarah went to Marks & Spencer. My only
contribution was to give my liver a rest for a couple of
nights.

I was expected at the crack of dawn for the first operating slot. With the gleeful prospect of having my naughty
bits on display for nurses I had worked with, I was up at
5.30 am and into the shower. I grabbed a couple of medical journals that had dropped through the letter box the
previous day, then Sarah drove me to town. After years of

putting this off, I experienced a mix of trepidation and relief as I stood in line at the reception desk, waiting to hand over my credit card. Then the ward itself was familiar to me. When we operated in the building on NHS waiting list initiative patients, they were housed here because it was next to the intensive care unit. From the consultants' names on the doors it now appeared to be a gynaecology ward. I knew my room well enough too. The only NHS ventricular assist device patient I had operated on in this hospital died here the night after leaving intensive care. The young woman had a huge cerebral bleed from an aneurysm in the brain. She was celebrating the relief from breathlessness and being able to lie flat again, to the delight of her husband and children who were there to visit her. It was pure serendipity that her surgeon was allocated that same haunted room ten years later.

Nurse Grace from Botswana came in to weigh me and record my vital signs. First the sphygmomanometer used to measure blood pressure didn't work. I just told her what my blood pressure normally was and suggested she added an increment for the anxiety I ought to be experiencing before surgery. Except that I felt no stress – I was more concerned before a haircut. Next Grace and I wandered out to a weighing machine in the corridor beside the nurses' station. That didn't seem to work either, so the poor girl became frantic with embarrassment. I told her it didn't matter, no one would ever look at my weight. With that I sat in the corner of the fateful room and flicked through the pages of the *British Medical Journal*. I always start at the back in the 'Jobs' section. I was still tempted by advertisements for a heart surgeon in Africa or the Middle East, where I could operate on children again. Indeed anywhere that valued technical skills and experience over fabricating appraisal forms or using that word 'reflection'.

Surprise, surprise. My eyes were immediately drawn to an article outlining the General Medical Council's new guidelines for 'reflection'. This kicked off with a statement: 'There is a strong public interest in doctors being able to reflect in an open and honest way.' Really? But so far, so good, because that's exactly what I've done in this book. They went on to say, 'Time should be made available for self-reflection and to reflect in groups.' Like group sex, I thought mischievously. By this point I was thinking about all the time I had wasted operating when I could have more profitably been reflecting. Perhaps Professor Cranston and I should enjoy a period of reflection together before my prostatectomy. We could reflect on all the operations the NHS couldn't do, such as my own, because surgeons were overwhelmed by bureaucratic crap.

What induces the General Medical Council to conclude that today's doctors are so thick that they need to be told how to think? Take this for a reflection. Virtually every heart surgery unit in the country has suffered a public scandal through working in highly pressured, inadequately staffed and poorly equipped facilities. Some of my post-operative deaths occurred because we didn't have consistent surgical or nursing teams – so-called 'failure to rescue' deaths, where the patients could have been saved by more effort and expertise. Few people can afford Oxford property, so we were inundated with temporary staff at enormous cost. When the General Medical Council claim that 'teams and groups improve patient care and service delivery when they are given opportunities to reflect together,' I say, 'Show me the bloody team and we'll find something to reflect upon.' Something other than 'You just fucking killed my patient.'

It was at this point that a monosyllabic Romanian doctor came in to take blood. 'I need to take some blood,' was all he said, but he did it skilfully by finding the vein first jab. And he knew to remove the tourniquet before extracting the needle so I didn't bruise or bleed. He then produced the consent form and told me to sign it, which I was happy to do. I was spared the dismal recital of potential complications that normally makes any sane patient run a mile.

As the efficient young man turned to leave, I said, 'Please tell Professor Cranston that I don't want any blood transfusion.' Then, tempting fate, I added, 'If I suffer a fatal stroke during surgery I'm happy to be an organ donor.' Altruistic to the end, but he didn't hear me so the gesture was wasted. With the introduction of 'presumed' consent in contrast to voluntary donation, I've since reconsidered that. It's a throwback to the body-snatching era.

I was still reading in my white theatre gown when Oliver Dyar the anaesthetist walked in. I had known Oliver for twenty years or more as one of the intensive care consultants who looked after my patients.

In his uncompromising manner he said, 'Steve, you could have a spinal anaesthetic and stay awake but frankly we don't want the interference. Nor will it get you out of here any quicker. So I'm putting you to sleep and will prescribe some pain medicine for afterwards. See you in a few minutes.'

That brief encounter was just what I wanted from the person responsible for keeping me both asleep and alive. I had no appetite for sycophantic compassion, empathy or any other emotional crap that had no bearing on the outcome of my operation. I had a bit of a phobia about waking up during the proceedings but was not going to insult him by mentioning it. Minutes later I wandered off to the operating theatre in my Marks & Spencer slippers and dressing gown. I jumped onto the trolley and stared at the ceiling, then, with a sharp needle prick in the back of my hand, I lapsed into unconsciousness. Anaesthetic in, lights out.

The squeeze of a functioning blood pressure cuff on my right arm roused me an hour or so later, and I emerged as if from fog in an unfamiliar place. I was staring across the recovery room that I used to look into from the operating theatre corridor, but it took me a while to work that out. There were conversations going on in the distance, then a question close by that seemed to be directed at me.

'How are you feeling?'

This was my recovery nurse in her purple dress. By reflex I groped down under the blanket at the stiff pipe emerging from my bladder. In doing so I yanked on the drip tubing, displacing the cannula in the back of my left hand and making it sting. This dragged me to my senses, shifting focus away from the nurse's legs. Fluid was pouring into my bladder from a gigantic plastic container, then it flushed out again to the drainage bag – crystal clear in, bright pink out. I felt that there couldn't be much bleeding, otherwise it would have been darker. Also there was no empty blood bag on the drip stand, so I assumed the operation had gone well. A deep sense of euphoria now suffused me. After ten years of misery I had finally summoned up the courage to sort myself out. And so far, it was less disagreeable than I'd expected.

By 2 pm I had talked with my family to confirm my survival and was back in the haunted room. Bored already, I began sifting through the journals again. I found another article in the *British Medical Journal* in its regular 'The Big Picture' section. The piece was entitled 'After a near decade's wait, a patient appeals for a donor heart' – his second, apparently – which could only have been written about the NHS. Allegedly, this man had been on a heart transplant waiting list at home for all that time. Now consider that the only patients proven to derive survival benefit after a heart transplant are those already in hospital on powerful drugs or circulatory support devices. So the title should have been 'Man celebrates 10 years of survival by avoiding a heart transplant'. But don't let's worry about facts or evidence. This was simply an emotional appeal for more organ donors when a rational argument to introduce ventricular assist devices would have been more appropriate. Take one from the shelf, stitch it into the failing heart and switch on the controller.

Symptoms gone, life extended, no dead person required.

I tossed the journal away and turned to the *Bulletin of the Royal College of Surgeons*. Oh shit! There was a paper entitled 'Surgeons' personalities and surgical outcomes', which explored the relationship between heart surgeons' personality types and their mortality rates. The punch line was that heart surgeons differ from the general population by being more extrovert, but that introverts have lower death rates than extroverts. Bloody obvious, I'd have said. Extroverts don't agonise about which patients to operate on or cherry pick to protect their results and reputations. What's more, introversion and a high level of conscientiousness were recognised as a recipe for stress and burnout. It transpired that the authors sent a questionnaire described as 'the most parsimonious and comprehensive model of normal adult personality' to all 261 consultant heart surgeons in the UK, then endeavoured to match these with their so-called 'risk-adjusted mortality rates' collected by the Society for Cardiothoracic Surgeons. The five characteristics examined were conscientiousness and openness, which I hope all doctors have; agreeableness and extroversion, which surgeons usually have; and lastly neuroticism, a feature of introverts from the outset.

Just ninety-six diligent individuals replied, and mortality statistics were available for only fifty-three of them. In reality, the authors of the paper had analysed information from a conscientious, self-selected one-fifth of the population, then derived the conclusion that those with the highest personality scores for openness killed more patients. On the basis of these curious findings, they concluded that the selection process for surgeons should admit more introverts. Yet we all know that extroverts made heart surgery possible in the first place when the introverts and neurotics were too stressed to continue. By now I was losing the will to live. In the two years since I stopped operating, 40 per cent of newly qualified heart surgeons had allegedly been suspended from practice – it was easy to see why.

The *Bulletin*'s next article – 'Surgery and emotional health' – didn't exactly inspire me with confidence either. It covered a series of Royal College of Surgeons workshops on 'stress, burnout and bullying', then 'anxiety, doubt and grief', followed by 'compassion and sympathy'. These touchy-feely events were undoubtedly attended by the introverts, while their extrovert colleagues stayed in the operating theatre boosting the body count. In a 'breakout discussion' focusing on 'recommendations for change', delegates to the event stressed that 'hospitals needed to make surgeons and their teams feel valued and appreciated, and help their staff develop supportive working relationships'. Poor paranoid, introverted surgeons. How things have changed in this business. I didn't belong anymore.

I mention these articles only because they provide a barometer on the prevailing attitudes among the surgical profession today. Fewer operations, more talking about it. For me this was Women's Institute coffee-morning stuff, just the ticket for the mandatory 'professional development' folder that we were all meant to compile for the

General Medical Council. It came as something of a relief that it was now time for Cranston to visit and tell me how he empathised with my prostate gland as chunks of it were tossed into the bin.

My whole career had been focused on repairing the sickest hearts at the highest risk, while avoiding nervous breakdowns about their owners. Sarah had done the same in her A&E departments. For us it was the patients who were important, not ourselves. Neither of us belonged in this modern medical world of introspection, reflection and compassion fatigue. My old friend Dr Cooley had just died in Houston, and I couldn't help thinking what he would have said about all this touchy-feely stuff. Of course, many would rejoice that the swashbuckling days of the flashing blade were over, maintaining that operations were meant to be boring and routine. What had we done to educate the public about our world when even the *British Medical Journal* considered a ten-year wait for a heart transplant to be believable?

That evening, nurse Sarah brought in a bottle of South African merlot to cheer me up. I was drinking red and pissing out rosé, but for the first night in years I wouldn't have to jump out of bed four or five times to pass water. A chatty night nurse came in with the evening drug round, so I turned off the lights and abandoned the journals for the evening's television soaps. Five minutes of *Casualty* had me reaching for the vomit bowl – or perhaps it was the dose of morphine that did that? In truth I wasn't feeling in any pain whatsoever, but was interested to be on the receiving end of an opioid shot just once in my life.

Merlot and morphine on a Saturday night. What could be better than that? Goodnight mundane reality, hello La La Land.

Whatever delights I hoped to derive were a far cry from what followed. That fiendish amygdala of mine spewed out a series of terrible medical memories into my cerebral cortex, so it was flashback time all over again. The ghosts of the departed popped by to visit their surgeon in hospital – my special patients, those I'd come to know too well, got too close to. A parade of battery-powered phantoms floated across the ceiling with turbines in their chest and electric plugs in their heads. Before this miracle of modern technology they had all been dying from heart failure, swollen with fluid, breathless after the slightest exertion, unable to lie flat or leave the house. They took their chance with me for a new life. They were the pulseless people.

For some it worked out well, for others it didn't. The former occupant of my bed appeared with bitterness in her eyes, blood spraying from her ears and nose as she darted across the room screeching that she should never have consented to it. Floating through the window came that nice chap for whom the drill bit went too deep, his skull thinner than we'd anticipated for such a big man. The brain surgeons removed the blood clot compressing his brain but he was too weakened by heart failure to recover. Pneumonia took him, but tonight he thanked me for our efforts. The phantom postman had been recovering at home when he tripped in the kitchen and struck his head. The paramedics found him unresponsive, cold on

the floor without a pulse, so they took him to the mortuary. But it was winter and all my turbine-pump patients
were pulseless, so I was really uneasy about it all. Yet his
ghost was pleased to see me and presented me with a box
containing his own struggling heart flapping around like
a wet fish.

The next pair were good friends and arrived together
straight through the closed door. Scotsman Jim was playing a lament on his bagpipes. His operation had been
shown throughout the world on the BBC's *Your Life in
Their Hands*. Two years later, at Christmas, he left home
without a spare battery, and when the pump's low-power
alarm sounded he had just twenty minutes to get back
and plug it in. He never made it.

Pulseless Peter was a religious man who had counselled
the others about life on a battery before their surgery. He
was the pioneer, the first patient in the world to be fitted
with a permanent turbine pump and the startling electric
plug in his skull. We became close friends, and he raised
money to buy pumps for other patients in his situation.
He would say, 'Life on a battery isn't normal life, but it's
better than the alternative.' And Lucky Jim would testify
to that. Although they were not yet sixty, both of them
had been turned down for a transplant, emotionally
devastating at the time.

On this particular night, the spectre of Peter was as
cheerful as ever because he loved to be with kindred spirits. He jovially referred to himself as 'Frankenstein's
monster' and secretly called me 'Driller Killer'. He always
promised to come back to haunt me, and I deeply regret-

ted being out of the country when he needed me most. After almost eight years of 'extra life' on the pump, Peter was by far the longest survivor with any type of artificial heart. His unnecessary death was a tragic debacle. When he suffered a profuse nose bleed, his one poorly function-ing kidney packed up, the local hospital declined to dial-yse him and I was uncontactable in Japan, so he joined Jim across the great divide. I was certain that he and his artificial heart could have lived beyond ten years, a land-mark a couple of my subsequent patients in other coun-tries have now achieved.

Merlot and morphine brought these tragic episodes back to me and, although the hallucinations were self-ter-minating, as usual I endured a long, restless night staring at the ceiling, unable to move, encumbered by the rhyth-mically pulsating anti-thrombosis leggings, transfixed by the irrigation system up my penis and tethered by the drip like a dog on a lead. Night nurse came in periodically to measure my blood pressure and for a while I thought she was part of the flashback. She looked at me strangely in the morning, so I wondered what I might have said to her. She'd been the only one without a wire cable emerging from her skull.

By Sunday morning the fluid coming out of my blad-der was almost clear, and following the previous day's fasting I was ravenously hungry. Now rational, I guessed that low blood sugar was the third element of the trio that had fuelled my hallucinations – the two M's, with added hypoglycaemia. Could that be reproduced, I wondered? Could I summon them all back for another phantom outpatient clinic? It was fascinating being deranged, and I could see why some people took drugs regularly.

I demolished the private hospital's full English breakfast, and sheepishly asked for kippers and toast as an encore. Then the nursing sister in charge that morning came in at the beginning of her shift, presumably having been told that I was delirious – or hilarious, perhaps. I told her I wanted this stiff pipe out of my prick as soon as possible, and emphasised the fact by extracting my own intravenous cannula and handing it to her. Off she went to call Professor Cranston. The morning sun shone through the curtains and I decided I'd had quite enough of being a patient. I knew the score. Bleeding stopped, catheter out, make sure I could piss, then home to my private nurse. Bugger three more days of paying for a haunted room and being treated like a recidivist.

I was working out how to dispense with the bladder catheter when sister came back.

'Professor Cranston says I can remove it if the washout is clear,' she said.

'Good. Let's get on with it.' I added that if I was still bleeding twenty-four hours after the surgery, I wanted my money back.

'But don't you even think about going home,' she said. 'It's far too soon for that.'

Being treated like a naughty child made up my contrary mind. Tomorrow the hospital would be full of people I'd once worked with, and I didn't want the whole of Oxford tuning in to my private parts.

Sister scrubbed her hands and slipped on rubber gloves with a determination that I found quite sinister – and suggestive. She aspirated water from the retaining balloon inside my bladder, then dragged the catheter out of me with a degree of mischief she could barely conceal, as if to say, 'Take some of that!' Blood clots that looked like purple seaweed and the odd fragment of prostate slid out with the balloon, followed by a dribble of fresh blood. This left me wondering, what if I went into retention now? How easy would it be to negotiate a catheter back through that raw space? I drank every drop of liquid in the room to build up a head of pressure before attempting the inaugural piss through my replumbed urinary tract. Then I paced the corridors in my spanking-new dressing gown and slippers, waiting for the urge to come.

At that point Oliver Dyar made his customary post-operative visit, a civilised and welcome gesture, which served to divert attention from my ragged urethra. More to the point, he was perturbed to hear of my intention to leave. Minutes later, David received a text message: 'OMG, he is going to go home.'

When the urge did finally arrive, I returned to my private facilities with an uncharacteristic sense of trepidation. Frankly, I expected it to hurt like hell the first time. And so it did, but the discomfort was surpassed by the sheer delight of pissing like a horse. So much so that I overshot considerably and had to mop it up. By the time the professor arrived at midday I was packed and ready to leave, quite possibly a record early discharge for a surgical prostatectomy. But I wouldn't contemplate another sleepless night in the hospital at considerable expense.

David was relaxed about it, like he is about most things as he heads for retirement. We live in close proximity, so he could always nip round if I got into trouble. I did continue to pass blood and clots for a couple of days, but this was trivial compared with the dramatic relief of obstruction and the salvage job for my kidneys. I just wished that I'd had it done years earlier.

Illness is as frightening for surgeons as it is for anyone else. Perhaps more so, given what we know. To quote one notable newspaper article, 'The only black mark against the NHS is its poor record in keeping people alive.' The main problem is that the service was launched as a nationalised industry designed to equalise access but not to maximise efficiency. I don't mind that myself, and my family has never received any preferential treatment – as occurs in other industries – but I do care when we can't get any treatment at all. The misery surrounding the seventieth anniversary of the NHS finally dispensed with that crass political deception: 'Our system is the envy of the world.' It simply isn't.

We lag behind other good healthcare systems in everything except economic stringency. We begin with higher infant mortality rates and continue through to poor outcomes for cancer and heart attacks. The most comprehensive report on cancer survival ever produced was published by *The Lancet* in 2018. This showed the NHS to be forty-seventh out of fifty-six countries for pancreatic cancer survival, forty-sixth for stomach cancer and forty-fifth for ovarian cancer, and that we lagged behind Latvia, Romania, Turkey and Argentina. Estimates suggest that 10,000 cancer deaths could be prevented each year if we were only average.

All this is not because our surgeons, doctors or nurses are poor. Quite the opposite. In general, they are talented, hardworking and care about the people they treat. Cut out the bureaucracy and regulatory crap, and they might be more productive. In better-functioning healthcare systems there are many more doctors, higher nurse–patient ratios and vastly shorter delays to assessment and treatment. There are more scanners, and lifesaving drugs and equipment are introduced in a timely fashion whatever their cost. Moreover, such systems are not subject to political ping-pong.

I have experienced all this myself in hospitals throughout Europe and the United States. My own doctor nephews have been working happily in Australia, while we offer Australian doctors golden handshakes to come here. But they don't. Only doctors from poor countries want to work in the NHS, and it shows. We are busy trying to attract medical and nursing staff from Asia and Africa, but these countries need them at home. The time has come for a radical rethink.

Better healthcare systems are not managed by the state, which regards more patients, procedures and technology as a burden. When emphasis remains on patient care not cost containment, other countries don't have to pay out £5 billion each year to settle medical negligence claims nor choose to ration treatment for osteoarthritis, hernias or varicose veins just because they are not life-threatening. Better healthcare systems don't have to discontinue all of their elective surgery for a month because of so-called seasonal pressures, as if winter were an unexpected event. What the NHS offered me, still a busy doctor with decades of service, was a one-year wait for surgery, during which time I'd have needed a urinary catheter and a plastic bag full of urine with me perpetually. No small wonder that Britain is the third-worst of eighteen Western countries in preventing avoidable deaths.

Yet no one has the guts to dismantle or reform this tarnished treasure for fear of being cast into political oblivion. You would have thought the serial horror stories and scandals that emerge daily – even from our best hospitals – would plant a red flag in the field. Labour hopes that the Conservatives will propose European or Australian funding models, just so they can attack them for deviating towards privatisation, while for that same reason the Tories studiously avoid any meaningful reform and simply sing the same tired old song. We are putting in billions of pounds to transform the NHS, but no one ever notices where this money goes or what it achieves. So we – the workers within the system – remain disillusioned. Neil Moat, the great cardiac surgeon who took stock of Sarah's labour when I was operating, retired prematurely from the Brompton to become medical director of a large pharmaceutical company in California. When I unexpectedly bumped into him in a café, he said, 'I just couldn't take any more of the NHS.'

The sad thing is that those of us at the sharp end did want the NHS to be the best. I had absolutely no interest in private practice throughout my whole career. I did original research, wrote scientific papers and published numerous textbooks, all to fly the flag for the NHS on the global stage. Surgeons gravitated to Oxford simply to learn how we could be so productive with so few resources. But the system couldn't give a toss. At sixty-eight I was threatened by the medical director with being 'sent off' because my Personal Development Plan for 'Revalidation' was not up to scratch. Reflect on that, General Medical Council. What was there to foster my 'emotional health' that the Royal College of Surgeons seem so keen on?

My truncated admission to the private sector made me think about what I most valued in a healthcare system. My first concern, whether in England or Africa, has to be access to treatment. Access is allegedly free in the NHS, but remember that we all – or most of us – pay for it in taxes. When we are sick we have four choices. First, an average wait of two weeks for an appointment with a GP. Next, a demoralising struggle through a questionnaire with the barefoot doctors on the 111 help line that's strictly focused on 'Do you need an ambulance soon, in four hours, or perhaps never?' Alternatively, you can go to a pharmacy for that critical opinion on your sick baby. And finally, you join the long queue of walking wounded in an A&E department, only to be dismissed as a time-waster and directed back to that GP's waiting list again. I've tried all of this for my family. Being pushed from pillar to post, the only thing that worked was to turn up at a hospital and join the queue. The primary care system has abrogated all responsibility for out-of-hours care, and clearly the hospital emergency services can't cope with the day-to-day service that the public demands. No surprises there then.

For myself, when I became far too worried to go through any of this, I phoned a friend – but the British public don't have that luxury. Should they be diagnosed with cancer, they have to endure a statutory and terrifying waiting time for treatment that's decided by politicians, not doctors. When I trained in America, anyone who needed heart surgery or an operation for cancer would have it that same week, as long as they had insured themselves, but when I went to Oxford many poor souls waited for more than a year for their operation – and some died on the waiting list. We called that 'cost containment'.

This leads nicely on to the subject of timely intervention – getting on with the investigations so that everyone knows what needs to be done, then receiving the prescribed treatment. Take a patient referred with anginal chest pain and a positive exercise test. Everyone knows that they have coronary artery disease, but they first wait months to see a cardiologist in the outpatient department, then there's another protracted delay for the coronary angiogram that dictates the appropriate treatment, then another hold-up to consult a cardiac surgeon, only to be told about an endless surgical waiting list. All of this while suffering from persistent symptoms, perpetual anxiety and the risk of premature death. How can the

British public tolerate this? It amounts to clinical negligence by the State.

In my last few years as a surgeon, many patients were subject to multiple cancellations before admission to hospital or even on the day of their operation, often because there were no available ward beds. Similarly, operated patients could not leave the intensive care unit through lack of ward beds – a vicious cycle of lousy management. Some of my patients were even discharged home directly from intensive care. Many of the elderly or sicker patients could not be discharged home because there was no one to look after them. Germany has 1,500 specialist rehabilitation hospitals, some with several hundred beds, so the same issues simply cannot occur. The NHS has none. Our patients are left to languish in their acute hospital beds, with serious adverse effects. Surgical patients and those recovering from stroke, head injury or heart attack lose up to 10 per cent of their leg muscle mass after ten days of inactivity, which in itself is equivalent to ten years of the aging process. So I am now working to build a 'state of the art' rehabilitation hospital in Oxford to maximise activity in the pressurised acute beds.

As patients we all need confidence in those designated to treat us. So how do the repeated hospital scandals, fuelled by the government and relished by the media, help us with all that? Bristol, Stafford, Gosport – names that linger in the memory, but the bureaucrats bear the responsibility, not those working at the coal face. At the root of these scandals, systems were at fault, not individuals. When I had my operation I wanted doctors with skill, experience and honesty to look after me – and I favour lucky surgeons that can get away with the unpredictable. While I value privacy and confidentiality, had I been having a more serious operation I really wouldn't have wanted to be invisible in a single room. Even with continuous remote monitoring, there needs to be someone watching – and usually there isn't. Nurses are far too busy to sit and watch monitor screens, so having staff and other patients in view is reassuring.

So where do empathy and compassion come into it? For me, they simply didn't matter. What I needed was to feel safe. And as we well know, our business-like NHS staff honestly don't have the time for the touchy-feely stuff. Some prostate surgery for cancer is done with robots. Surprisingly, robots don't manifest sympathy or compassion, although they could be programmed to say, 'I feel your pain, I feel your pain,' over and over again while digging out the bad bits.

Yet there are times and situations when kindness helps. Back to the *British Medical Journal*, which recently published an article entitled 'The difference that compassionate care makes'. The following were the thoughts of a lady professor in Denmark whose baby suffered then died from an inherited genetic disorder. She wrote:

> Empathetic care can support patients' and relatives' attempts to understand and cope with the inexplicable – be it the death of a child, the diagnosis of an illness, or one of the many other experiences that bring us into contact with healthcare systems.

The author described meeting 'incredibly caring doctors', but also 'hurried and disengaged doctors who appeared unable to truly see the patient – my son – and myself'.

I would argue that such differentiation is false. The strong likelihood is that the doctors she saw were all caring people, but the impression they left depended upon their workload at the time. NHS GPs have eight minutes to greet, diagnose and treat their patients, then write the records. How does that work for those with mental health issues? They may see fifty people in one day. Given such taxing circumstances, their focus has to remain on not making a mistake. It's the same story on the wards, in the A&E department and in the operating theatre – pressure-cooker environments with shortages of staff in every discipline, except management. Maybe the NHS should appoint 'compassion and empathy' managers, because time-pressured clinical staff have to maintain their objectivity, and cannot possibly delve into the hopes and fears of their patients, as perhaps they did in the good old days.

What I regret most about the economic expediency of the NHS is that clinical efficiency and productivity detract from aspects of the doctor–patient relationship, and that needs to be recognised. It takes a particular mindset to deal with the spectre of death on a daily basis, which is why those psychological surveys demonstrate a surprising preponderance of psychopathic tendencies in surgeons, children's cancer doctors and psychiatrists. I rarely lost a child, but when I did I had to walk away from it. I couldn't keep putting myself in the parents' shoes, otherwise I wouldn't come to work the following day. That is what burnout is all about. It was the difference between John Gibbon, the inventor of the heart–lung machine, and John Kirklin, who made that incredibly daunting equipment work for patients. When Gibbon lost a series of children, he gave up. Kirklin didn't, nor did Lord Brock. I had the great privilege of following in their pioneering footsteps. Sadly, no one else will have that freedom now.

So, if I may, please let me conclude with a quote from George Orwell:

Autobiography is only to be trusted when it reveals something disgraceful. A man who gives a good account of himself is probably lying, since any life when viewed from the inside is simply a series of defeats.

I understand just what he meant by that.

acknowledgements

SUCH WAS MY FASCINATION with the quest to operate meaningfully within the heart that I wrote a comprehensive textbook on the subject called *Landmarks in Cardiac Surgery* (1997). While researching the intrepid pioneers I made contact with many of them, who in their twilight years were keen to record their memories. These were great characters from both sides of the Atlantic who risked, and often experienced, a death every operating day. As I gradually came to meet them all in person they proved to be a great inspiration for me. Their advice? Always search for a better way. Our specialty still has a long way to go.

My own career began in some of Britain's finest institutions, which included the Royal Brompton Hospital, Addenbrooke's Hospital in Cambridge, then the Hammersmith Hospital and Royal Postgraduate Medical School, and the Hospital for Sick Children at Great Ormond Street. Following training in Britain and the United States, I spent the rest of my career amid the dreaming spires of Oxford. Irrespective of the moans,

groans and frustration expressed in this book, I unreserv-
edly rank the Oxford University Hospitals and their dedicated staff as among the finest in Europe. Those who 'toil
at the coal face' define a hospital, not the buildings, politicians or the NHS itself. So I would like to extend my
boundless gratitude to all the colleagues who supported
my patients and me in the office, on the wards, in the
operating theatres and the intensive care unit, during
good times and bad, joyful and sad. Together we achieved
world firsts, spectacular saves and notable changes to the
way cardiac surgery is practised globally. Innovation was
born of necessity – or lack of funds, to be brutally honest.
Of course, the NHS turned a blind eye to our achievements, but high honours from the United States, Russia
and Japan more than compensated for that. Forgive the
boasting – and a few swear words in the text, which I use
for emphasis but blame on the head injury! I seldom
swore at work.

Cardiac surgery relies upon finely honed team work
and round-the-clock care, which would have been impossible without the fine international fellows who trained
with me in Oxford, then returned to be eminent surgeons
in their own countries. Training is what we should be
doing, not poaching overseas staff to fill spaces made by
the deficiencies in what many claim to be a first world
healthcare system. While we clinicians rarely acknowledge the fact, I also appreciated the efforts of some dedicated hospital managers who went out of their way to
help rather than hinder us. In short, these great hospitals
and professional relationships defined my career in a way

that can never be repeated, thanks to 'modernisation'. To use a well-worn phrase, 'They don't make them like that anymore.'

Born within weeks of its inception in 1948, my whole working life was spent supporting our precious NHS. But should it once more aspire to provide first-rate treatment, it must invest more in staff and equipment and less in bureaucracy and committees to promote cost containment. Contemporary medicine and surgery are inordinately expensive. As an 'off-the-shelf' alternative to a heart transplant, the implantable rotary heart pumps I pioneered cost more than a Ferrari. Other European countries use them, so Britain needs to learn from more successful healthcare systems right now before it is too late.

I would like to express my thanks to the doctors, named patients and their relatives who were happy, enthusiastic even, for me to write about them. Others, from early in my career, are sadly no longer with us and their circumstances have been adjusted sufficiently for them not to be recognisable.

Finally, what I valued most in life was the unwavering love and support from my family. It is an understatement to explain that I was never easy to live with. I left the house before dawn, worked late, travelled too much, then was knackered when I returned home. After leaning over an operating table all day I would tell the wife, 'Sorry I'm so tired. My back's bad and the front's not so good either.' But everyone appreciated my efforts to save lives. That is why I wrote both *Fragile Lives* and *The Knife's Edge*, so that they may eventually understand who I was, and what I tried to achieve during those years. Special people, my family.

glossary

acute heart failure: the left ventricle fails rapidly and
cannot sustain sufficient blood flow to the body. The
lungs then fill with fluid. Usually caused by
myocardial infarction or viral myocarditis and has a
high mortality rate. *See also* shock.

angina: crushing pain in the chest, neck and left arm due
to limitation of blood flow to heart muscle in coronary
artery disease. Typically comes on during exercise. If it
comes on at rest it may warn of a heart attack.

angiogram: cardiological investigation where a long
catheter is passed through the blood vessels into the
heart. This allows blood pressure to be measured in
the cardiac chambers and dye to be injected to
visualise the coronary arteries or aorta.

aorta: large, thick-walled artery that leaves the left
ventricle then branches to supply the whole body. The
first small branches are the coronary arteries, which
supply blood to the heart itself.

aortic stenosis: narrowing of the aortic valve at the
outlet of the left ventricle, restricting blood flow

around the body. Can be caused by a congenital anomaly or degeneration in old age.

arteries: the blood vessels that convey blood to the organs and muscles of the body.

atrioventricular canal: congenital heart defect where there is a continuous hole between the collecting (atria) and pumping (ventricles) chambers, and the mitral and tricuspid valves fail to form properly.

blood pressure: pressure within the large arteries. Normally measured by a cuff and stethoscope or a cannula inserted into an artery. Normal blood pressure is around 120/80 mm Hg. The higher figure is when the left ventricle contracts; the lower, when it relaxes.

bridge to recovery: the process whereby a ventricular assist device is used to sustain the circulation and rest an acutely failing heart pending recovery from a reversible condition. If the heart does not recover, a limited-duration pump can be replaced by a long-term implanted device.

bridge to transplant: the process whereby a ventricular assist device is used to prevent death from heart failure until a donor heart can be found. At the time of transplant the pump and diseased heart are both removed.

cannula: a plastic tube inserted into the heart or a blood vessel to carry blood or fluid.

cardiac tamponade: a condition that occurs when blood or fluid accumulates within the pericardial sac under pressure, preventing the heart from filling.

cardioplegia: a cold (4°C) clear or blood-based solution infused into the coronary arteries to stop and protect the heart in a flaccid state during surgery with the heart–lung machine. Usually contains a high concentration of potassium. At the end of the repair the heart is re-animated by restoring normal coronary blood flow.

cardiopulmonary bypass (CPB): process whereby the patient's blood is diverted away from the heart and lungs for the duration of the surgical repair. Contact of the patient's blood with the synthetic surfaces in the pump-oxygenator system elicits an inflammatory response. This limits the safe duration of blood–foreign surface interaction. The longer the procedure, the more damaging is the whole-body inflammatory response.

congenital heart disease: heart deformity that the patient is born with (e.g. atrial septal defect, ventricular septal defect, dextrocardia).

coronary artery disease: gradual narrowing of the coronary arteries by atheroma. These fatty, cholesterol-based plaques are prone to rupture when they suddenly occlude the vessel, which then clots (coronary thrombosis).

crash call: call for a resuscitation team of doctors and nurses.

CT scan: X-ray-based three-dimensional imaging of the chest and heart. By adding contrast medium, the coronary arteries can be shown in detail.

Dacron: a woven fabric used to make vascular tube grafts and heart patches.

defibrillate: electric shock of between 10 and 20 joules used to restore normal heart rhythm during the disordered rhythm of ventricular fibrillation.

deoxygenated blood: bluish blood leaving the tissues and returning to the right heart, now low in oxygen and carrying carbon dioxide to be expelled by the lungs. *See also* oxygenated blood.

diastole: relaxation and filling phase of the ventricles.

direct vision: to see within the heart in order to conduct a surgical repair.

distal anastomosis: join between a coronary bypass graft and the target coronary artery.

echocardiogram: non-invasive ultrasound examination of the heart chambers.

electrocautery: the electrical instrument used to cut through tissues and simultaneously coagulate blood vessels to stop bleeding.

endocarditis: bacterial infection that can destroy the heart valves.

endotracheal tube: tube in the windpipe through which to ventilate a patient.

exsanguinate: bleed to death.

heart–lung machine: circuit outside the body to keep the patient alive while the heart is stopped for repair. Contains a mechanical blood pump and a short-term (lasting hours) complex gas exchange mechanism known as the oxygenator (artificial lung). Other pumps are used for suction of blood into the reservoir and for delivery of cardioplegia fluid to stop the heart.

HeartMate left ventricular assist device: an obsolete large pulsatile implantable pump widely used for bridge to transplant in the 1990s. The first device to be implanted on a permanent basis. Thoratec went on to produce a successful rotary blood pump for permanent use.

heart transplant: removal of the patient's diseased and failing heart, then replacement with an organ from a brain-dead donor.

heart valve replacement: removal of a diseased heart valve, then replacement with a prosthetic valve. Prosthetic valves can be biological (e.g. pig's valve) or mechanical (e.g. pyrolytic carbon tilting disc valves).

homograft bank: department that collects and processes human heart valves and blood vessels donated by the deceased for use in patients.

iliac fossa: part of the lower abdominal wall beneath the umbilicus.

inferior vena cava: *see* vena cava.

intubation: the process of inserting the endotracheal tube into the patient for ventilation.

left atrium: collecting chamber for blood returning to the heart from the lungs. The blood then passes through the mitral valve into the left ventricle. *See also* right atrium.

left ventricle: powerful, thick-walled conical chamber that pumps blood through the aortic valve and around the body. *See also* right ventricle.

left ventricular assist device (LVAD): mechanical blood pump to maintain the circulation and rest the ventricles when the heart fails catastrophically. The cannulas are inserted into the chambers of the heart. There are inexpensive temporary external devices suitable for several weeks of support in acute heart failure (e.g. CentriMag or Berlin Heart). The small, implantable but very expensive high-speed rotary blood pumps (e.g. Jarvik 2000) can be used for as long as ten years in chronic heart failure. As such, the long-term LVADs offer an off-the-shelf alternative to heart transplantation.

metabolic derangement: consequence of poor tissue blood flow. Arteries to the muscles clamp down and the tissues produce lactic acid and other toxic metabolites.

mitral stenosis: narrowing of the mitral valve between left atrium and left ventricle caused by rheumatic fever. Flow through the valve is restricted, causing breathlessness and chronic fatigue.

mitral valve: valve between the left atrium and ventricle. Named after a bishop's mitre.

oxygenated blood: bright red blood saturated with oxygen and pumped around the body by the left ventricle. *See also* deoxygenated blood.

perfusionist: technician who controls the heart–lung machine and ventricular assist devices.

pericardium: fibrous sac that surrounds the heart. Can be used as patch material in the heart. Calf pericardium is used to make bioprosthetic heart valves.

pulmonary artery: large, thin-walled vessel that carries blood from the right ventricle to the lungs.

reperfusion: the process whereby blood is allowed back into the coronary arteries and heart muscle following cardioplegia and cardiac arrest during surgery. The heart is re-animated and begins to beat again.

resident: trainee surgeon in the US, so-called because they live in the hospital.

rheumatic fever: autoimmune condition triggered by a streptococcus bacterial infection that damages the heart valves and joints. Very common cause of rheumatic valve disease in the pre-antibiotic era.

right atrium: collecting chamber for blood returning to the heart from the body via the veins. The blood then passes through the tricuspid valve into the right ventricle. *See also* left atrium.

right ventricle: crescent-shaped pumping chamber that propels blood through the pulmonary valve and to the lungs. *See also* left ventricle.

sharps bin: bin in which to deposit needles and scalpel blades after contact with blood.

shock: condition when the heart cannot continue to supply sufficient blood and oxygen to the tissues. Cardiogenic shock occurs after a heart attack. Haemorrhagic shock follows profuse bleeding of two litres or more.

tricuspid valve: valve between the right atrium and right ventricle.

valvotomy: surgical manoeuvre to dilate the narrowed orifice of an aortic or mitral valve.

veins: thinner-walled vessels that return blood to the heart.

vena cava: large vein entering the right atrium. The superior vena cava drains the upper part of the body; the inferior vena cava drains the lower half.